Clinical Supervision and Mentorship in Nursing

SECOND EDITION

Edited by

Tony Butterworth
Jean Faugier
Philip Burnard

Stanley Thornes (Publishers) Ltd

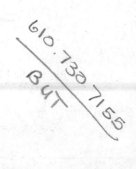

© 1992, 1998 Stanley Thornes (Publishers) Ltd

First published by Chapman & Hall in 1992

Reprinted in 1997 by:
Stanley Thornes (Publishers) Ltd
Ellenborough House
Wellington Street
CHELTENHAM
GL50 1YW
United Kingdom

Second edition 1998

98 99 00 01 02 / 10 9 8 7 6 5 4 3 2 1

A catalogue record for this book is available from the British Library.

ISBN 0 7487 3304 3

Typeset by Acorn Bookwork, Salisbury
Printed and bound in Great Britain by T.J. International Ltd., Padstow, Cornwall

Contents

Contributors   v

Introduction to second edition   ix

1 Clinical supervision as an emerging idea in nursing   1
       Tony Butterworth

2 The supervisory relationship   19
       Jean Faugier

3 The therapeutic use of self   37
       David Woods

4 Clinical supervision, stress management and social support   49
       Jerome Carson, Tony Butterworth and Katie Booth

5 Psychiatric nursing   66
       Phil Barker

6 Clinical supervision in sick children's nursing   81
       Barbara Elliott and Judith Ellis

7 Developing supervision in adult/general nursing   95
       Carol Marrow and Talib Yaseen

8 Clinical supervision in learning disabilities nursing   113
       Sandy Bering, Ross Brocklehurst and Michelle Teasdale

9 Child protection: health visiting and supervision   132
       Robert Nettleton

10 The supervision of health visiting practice: a continuing agenda
       for debate   153
       Sheila Twinn and Claire Johnson

11 Clinical supervision in district nursing   174
       Brian Pateman

12 Clinical supervision and community psychiatric nursing   189
       Peter Wilkin

13 Modelling excellence: the role of the consultant nurse 205
Steve Wright

14 'Supervision for life' 215
Tony Butterworth and Jean Faugier

15 Evaluation research in clinical supervision: a case example 220
Tony Butterworth

Index 233

Contributors

Phil Barker
Department of Psychiatry, Royal Victoria Infirmary, Newcastle-upon-Tyne
Chapter 5, Psychiatric nursing

Sandy Bering
Chester and Halton Community NHS Trust, Cheshire
Chapter 8, Clinical supervision in learning disability nursing

Katie Booth
Department of Nursing, The University of Liverpool, Liverpool
Chapter 4, Clinical supervision, stress management and social support

Ross Brocklehurst
The School of Nursing, Midwifery and Health Visiting, University of Manchester, Manchester
Chapter 8, Clinical supervision in learning disability nursing

Philip Burnard
School of Nursing Studies, University of Wales College of Medicine, Cardiff

Tony Butterworth
School of Nursing, Midwifery and Health Visiting, University of Manchester, Manchester
Chapter 1, Clinical supervision as an emerging idea in nursing
Chapter 4, Clinical supervision, stress management and social support
Chapter 14, 'Supervision for life'
Chapter 15, Evaluation research in clinical supervision: a case example

Jerome Carson
Institute of Psychiatry, London.
Chapter 4, Clinical supervision, stress management and social support

Barbara Elliott
School of Nursing, University of Hull, Hull
Chapter 6, Clinical supervision in sick children's nursing

Judith Ellis
Royal Preston Hospital, Fulwood, Preston
Chapter 6, Clinical supervision in sick children's nursing

Jean Faugier
NHS Executive North West, Warrington
Chapter 2, The supervisory relationship
Chapter 14, 'Supervision for life'

Claire Johnson
Department of Nursing Studies, The Chinese University of Hong Kong, Hong Kong
Chapter 10, The supervision of health visiting practice: a continuing agenda for debate

Carol Marrow
Furness General Hospital, Barrow-in-Furness
Chapter 7, Developing supervision in adult/general nursing

Robert Nettleton
Faculty of Arts, Science and Education, Bolton Institute of Higher Education, Bolton
Chapter 9, Child protection: health visiting and supervision

Brian Pateman
School of Nursing, Midwifery and Health Visiting, University of Manchester, Manchester
Chapter 11, Clinical supervision in district nursing

Michelle Teasdale
Chester and Halton Community NHS Trust, Cheshire
Chapter 8, Clinical supervision in learning disability nursing

Sheila Twinn
Department of Nursing, The Chinese University of Hong Kong, Hong Kong
Chapter 10, The supervision of health visiting practice: a continuing agenda for debate

Peter Wilkin
Taylor Street Clinic, Heywood
Chapter 12, Clinical supervision and community psychiatric nursing

Steve Wright
TENDA, Redmire, Mungrisdale, Cumbria
Chapter 13, Modelling excellence: the role of the consultant nurse

David Woods
School of Nursing, Midwifery and Health Visiting, University of Manchester, Manchester
Chapter 3, The therapeutic use of self

Talib Yaseen
Nursing and Operational Services, Furness General Hospital, Barrow-in-Furness
Chapter 7, Developing supervision in adult/general nursing

Introduction to second edition

The second edition of this book comes at a time when clinical supervision and mentorship are riding high on the research and service development agenda. Since publication of the first edition in 1992, the subject has been the focus of intense debate from clinicians, educators, researchers and policy-makers. The breadth of this debate demonstrates the way in which clinical supervision and mentorship has caught the imagination of people across the professions. It is most encouraging to note that it has remained largely in the hands of clinicians and those most directly involved in the delivery of care, which must be a testimony to its utility for practice.

This second edition has addressed some of the developments which have taken place in research and in education. The authors decided to continue to address the particular subject specialities in the profession and retain some of the 'introductory' flavour of the first edition, as it is quite clear that there are many staff still working on introducing it in their workplace.

We have started well, but there is still some way to go. The real development of clinical supervision and mentorship is only just beginning as services record and evaluate its impact on services in a wide range of specialities. Their accounts, which are reported in part in this book, will provide the testimony to how the professions use this valuable tool in practice. The ultimate goal is surely when clinical supervision and mentorship become 'unremarkable' and part of everyday practice.

Tony Butterworth
July 1998

Clinical supervision as an emerging idea in nursing

1

Tony Butterworth

The University of Manchester can lay some justifiable claim to having raised the debate on clinical supervision in the United Kingdom. In 1988, at its annual Good Practices in Community Nursing Conference, it was argued that some means of supporting safe professional practice should be offered and that 'community nurses and health visitors must investigate a means of providing clinical supervision' as it provided 'a well tested vehicle for evolutionary practice and should be the cornerstone for any profession which has person centred clinical involvement at its heart' (Butterworth, 1988).

For clinical services and university departments it is important to pursue these noble ideas through research endeavour, and we are beginning to share the product of sustained research and development activity. From tentative beginnings, the implementation of clinical supervision and the debate which surrounds it appears to have reached a peak in the last part of the millennium.

Nursing itself has undergone striking changes in the 1990s. New roles and structures, and demands for advanced practice have asked great things of nurses. Exciting times indeed, but the need to surround these new ways of working with safe supportive supervision and debate is just as important.

There are tensions which have yet to be resolved, not least of which is the very title 'clinical supervision'. There are those who take exception to the term clinical supervision, indeed the United Kingdom Central Council for Nursing, Midwifery and Health Visiting has extensively debated the point in its run-up to a final statement (UKCC, 1996). A confident, expert professional has little to worry about from being supervised. If the concern of clinical supervision is to sustain and develop professional practice, then its intentions are clearly honourable and not to be feared.

Doubts about being supervised most often relate to its potential to be abused as a system of unnecessary control and interference in professional autonomy. For the most part, clinical supervision is a practice-led activity, and when secured within this practice embrace, it is less likely to be abused.

There is growing evidence that other professions are beginning to explore the ideas which surround clinical supervision. Managers, senior medical staff and general practitioners are experimenting with what they call (somewhat confusingly for nurses) mentorship schemes. These schemes show some of the characteristics of clinical supervision, and there are points at which these matters can be explored through multi-disciplinary work.

An important debate lies in attempting to make judgements on the impact that clinical supervision has on patients and their families. Attempts are being made (more often through argument rather than action) to relate the impact of clinical supervision to patient outcome. These arguments at worst allow services not to implement clinical supervision, and at best suggest that while the importance of impacting on patient outcome is undeniable, absolutely everything else is subsumed by it, including the well-being of the workforce.

These attempts to link clinical supervision to patient outcome are not well advanced and, indeed, may prove so elusive and complex to construct in real life that no one will attempt them. Presently, what is more easy to demonstrate is the link between clinical supervision, work practices and the well-being of the workforce. This is in itself a worthy endeavour and its value should not to be underestimated.

Encouragingly, most developments in clinical supervision are being led by those with immediate practice experience and so the problem of theory being dislocated from practice may not be quite so problematic.

The growing literature on the subject of clinical supervision is encouraging. However, it is still useful to consider some of those influences which led nursing in this particular direction.

BEGINNINGS

In its attempt to gain independence and achieve mature self-determination, nursing has with varying degrees of success attempted to pull away from roots of origin which tie it, amongst other things, to the medical profession.

The nursing profession has moved a long way from seeing itself as a less well-prepared or educated assistant to the doctor, and has become increasingly aware that many roles within nursing and medicine mirror gender roles within society. Nursing could be said to contain a high proportion of expressive roles which carry little attendant power and responsibility. The cost of this lack of professional power is, of course, reflected in comparatively low financial reward. However, the consequences of being professionally less powerful and in seldom carrying overall responsibility for patient care have been manifested in low levels of risk-taking and accountability by nurses. Medicine, on the other hand, carries high material rewards and requires the exercise of power and responsibility, which is a common characteristic of male-dominated professions. Interestingly, however, whilst doctors cannot avoid overall responsibility, it is possible for them to diffuse the emotional cost of their role through the demands and consequences of working as 'scientists' and by delegation to nursing.

Nursing carries high emotional cost consequences which occasionally are difficult if not impossible to handle. Menzies (1960) describes vividly the effects of this emotional cost in relation to the organization of nursing as a social system striving to avoid inherent anxiety by the avoidance of the individual patient or colleague. It is the growing consciousness of the issues posed in the change from task-oriented nursing practice which has focused attention on the need for 'support' for the clinical nurse faced with dealing not simply with the patient's psychology, but also her own.

Attempts to de-medicalize nursing are to be found in the literature and are often posited as evidence of a new-found independence (Pearson, 1988). As these old ties are cut, it might be argued that there is a danger of nursing being left without a source of theoretical nourishment. Interestingly, it appears that the reverse is true, as new areas of contributory knowledge are described and receive explanation. The traditional underpinning influences of the curriculum base of nurse education have been the biological and medical sciences which carry both the kudos of having some 'scientific respectability' and also the inappropriateness and frustrations of reductionism. These constraints have been partially traded-off as nursing has moved towards the social sciences and looked for explanations from sociology, psychology and theories in education. In order to accommodate these changes, new ways of organizing and presenting nursing care have been established. Most notable of these has been the introduction of the nursing process. The nursing process is seen as a means of ordering nursing care while at the same time being sufficiently flexible to allow changes in theoretical influences and individualized care. Nurses have been urged to reconsider their work within categories which assess, plan and evaluate their work. The key difference in this approach is that it makes task-centred work a thing of the past, and recommends person-centred work with individualized planning as a means to action. Within the process approach, nurses have been urged to make closer and more meaningful relationships with patients and attend to the social, emotional and psychological requirements of people under their care. Unfortunately, less energy has been spent in helping nurses understand and work with the consequences of close interpersonal exchanges.

In tandem with the nursing process, theories of nursing have appeared which have produced descriptions and paradigms which might provide a base for nursing. The vehicle which takes these theoretical propositions to the clinical setting is the nursing process and within these theories nurses are again urged to 'form a relationship' with patients. Once again the consequences of doing so often receive little or no attention from the theoreticians. It follows that nursing has occasionally confused itself and more often alienated its medical and paramedical colleagues by throwing up new theories and action strategies which lay disputable and sometimes confusing territorial claims to new theories and actions which are themselves ill-defined.

As we have progressively removed the protective, if somewhat stifling, layers of professional management, nursing has become more visibly accountable for its work in the clinical setting. Equally it is important to recognize that the more exposed nurses have become to intimate nurse–patient relationships the weaker and more ill-defined have become their protective devices, devices which are not always enabling and have been so clearly identified by Menzies (1960) and Stockwell (1972). In shaking off the paternalist hand of medicine, the protection it provided has gone with it, and little has been done to replace it from within nursing itself. Although nursing has made great strides towards independence (Butterworth, 1990), the attraction of working in teams led by doctors is still evident, offering a paternalism which is more comforting than an independence which carries attendant responsibilities. Small wonder then that nurses show some dissonance about the unprotected opportunism which beckons and the shielded paternalism which frustrates. It is a contention of this book that models of clinical supervision in nursing will protect and improve upon clinical practice and give nursing the necessary support it needs to mature into independence.

The process of development is well under way. The accountability and responsibilities of nurses are becoming enshrined in recommendations from statutory bodies. In 1989 the English National Board for Nurses, Midwives and Health Visitors, in a paper *Preparation of Teachers, Practitioner/Teachers, Mentors and Supervisors in the context of Project 2000* (ENB, 1989), was one of the first to recognize an evolutionary change in the nurse–student if not nurse–patient relationship. It is suggested that 'those involved in teaching, facilitating others' learning, supervising and assessing, will need to have particular attributes and develop specific competencies'. However, the means to achieving this are less clearly defined. This paper was something of a milestone as it raised and debated a number of terms for the first time. Because of its particular remit, however, it was limited to the changing role of the educationalist and student and does not take the debate into the more general arena of practice. This is a pity, as qualified and experienced nurses are equally in need of similar consideration and it is a second contention of this book that clinical supervision is a model which must endure throughout professional life, thus providing a supportive as well as an educative purpose. An example of supportive supervision is postulated by Wright (1986) when he argues:

'It seems logical to assume that if nurses are to treat patients as human beings, then they in turn need to be treated in the same way by those who manage and educate them. If nurses, through reorganising their working patterns and permitting partnership with patients, are to have their traditional props pulled from under them, then they need help to find new ways of coping. Opportunities to share feelings, to express views and raise questions are essential; those in management positions at whatever level can provide the new props by an open, supportive and accepting style.'

A framework to allow continuous professional development has been provided by the United Kingdom Central Council in their report on post-registration and practice (UKCC, 1990). Its working group had as one of its terms of reference:

'to devise a coherent and comprehensive framework incorporating the standards and principles of education and practice beyond registration to meet the needs of patients and the health services.'

In response, the UKCC presents in its report a model of the continuum of practice and suggest that:

'a form of post-registration education must occur at least every three years – practitioners have no end point in their need to maintain and develop standards of practice.'

It should therefore be possible to devise a model of continuous supervision throughout professional life and accord with requirements of the professional body. The continuum of mentorship from student through clinical supervision to qualified professional becomes apparent.

MENTORSHIP

The role of mentor gained prominence particularly within educational programmes being developed within Project 2000. Not surprisingly this is territory already visited by American nurses. Darling (1984), one of the pioneers of mentorship in the United States, has gone so far as to devise a system for measuring mentorship potential (The Darling MMP2), and has outlined the characteristics of 'good mentors'. These include being:

- an envisioner: giving the learner a picture of what nursing can be like;
- a standard prodder: pushing the learner to achieve high standards;
- a challenger: making the learner look more closely at her skills and the decisions she makes.

Other writers also emphasize this active educational element. Peutz (1985) describes mentors as possessing several specific functions, including serving as teachers, sponsors, hosts, exemplars and counsellors. Mentors are seen as sharing their experience, thus teaching the best way of doing things, enhancing their protégées' skills and furthering their intellectual ability. One could be forgiven for thinking that this approach is quite a way from those less certain, more facilitative models traditionally employed in psychotherapy and social work. It is not surprising that nursing, a profession which finds itself uncomfortable with uncertainty, is attracted to models arrogant enough to claim that mentors or supervisors know the best way of doing things, and have it within their capabilities to enhance skills and further their intellectual development.

Such complex developments are better considered as a product of growth through interaction in a safe and stimulating relationship based on openness and trust, and are as much the responsibility and achievement of the supervisee as of the supervisor. To follow models of mentorship which see things being told to, done to and given to students is simply to mirror the process of clinical nursing in which things were done to patients without them being active in the partnership. Burnard (1989), advocating the role of mentor to district nurses, describes a paradigm proposed by Darling (1984) in which she identifies three aspects to the role of mentor – inspirer, investor and supporter – and suggests that, within the role of mentor, it is possible to model effective nursing practice. Such a proposition places this aspect of the role of mentor outside the role of traditional nurse educator in the United Kingdom. The nurse educator has often become deskilled through lack of practice contact and cannot therefore act as a model of good practice. This is not to criticize, rather to illustrate an evolution in the way that nurse educators have moved away from the practice setting. There have been a number of alternative suggestions, however, which see a role for a teacher/practitioner who might combine maintained clinical skills with a role of teacher (Jarvis and Gibson, 1985). Darling's second aspect of mentoring, 'investment', suggests that each learner has worth, and a measure of potential that can be encouraged, developed and refined in tandem with a mentor. This bears some comparison to a Rogerian view (Rogers, 1951) that for a relationship to achieve progress there must be warm positive unconditional regard, a proposition well-known to those involved in counselling. A Rogerian model has no strong base in nursing although the profession has flirted with it in recent times by encouraging nurses to make a 'nurse–patient relationship'. Equally, interpersonal skills have been explored in nursing curricula, although the means to acquiring them has not been without criticism.

The third part of the triangulation of mentorship is that of supporter. Burnard (1989) suggests that this requires the skills of active listening and empathy. One could hypothesize that to be raised as a student in a learning environment which encourages these skills will lead to qualified nurses who will foster similar therapeutic exchanges between nurses and patients.

There remains some work to be done on who might be the most suitable mentor 'material'. Such a demanding role obviously requires a competence over and above that of simply being able to function as a trained nurse. A number of concerned commentators in nursing have pointed out the need to be aware of the tremendous importance of choosing those who act as mentors and supervisors. Burnard (1988) highlights the likelihood that:

'the relationship between student and mentor also invokes transference, particularly as the mentor is already cast in the role of "expert" by the very fact that she is a mentor. All this suggests that mentors should be chosen very carefully. Who should be doing the choosing remains a question for debate.'

The work of mentors and supervisors in education has been the subject of research attention which has shed some light on the processes and good working practices of mentors and their students. One of the most comprehensive studies, funded by the English National Board was conducted by the Universities of London and Manchester (ENB, 1994).

In reporting on the ENB study, White (1996) suggests that a number of key points arose from this exploratory two-stage study on clinical supervision and Project 2000 students:

- confusion in the titles and functions of mentors led to competition with competing demands on mentor time;
- problems with educational support when staffing levels were low;
- students demonstrably thrive under sustained supervision.

Spouse (1996) reports on a longitudinal naturalistic study over four years and describes a number of key points from her work:

- learning in clinical practice works best when mentors develop a caring and trusting relationship with students;
- mentoring requires a match between learning need and available learning opportunities;
- staffing levels need to reflect the additional work required on the mentor's role.

Literature on the role of mentor is becoming the subject of scrutiny in other health-care professions and by managers, as they see value in the coaching and promoting role that a mentor carries for professional development after qualification and throughout professional life.

CLINICAL SUPERVISION

It has been suggested by Hill (1989) that people at work tend to think of their supervisors as authoritarian and that the whole concept of supervision is linked conceptually to an authority figure. This is a pity, because clinical supervision is much wider and more generous in its intentions. Peer support is often given as an example of supervision carried out by nurses, and most nurses would agree that it is done regularly on an informal basis, although few have constructed the opportunity to formalize peer support to the extent that can be found in nurse development units. An example of informal peer support is the 'tea break/tear break', often used as a way of letting colleagues share in stressful clinical experiences which have affected nurses in their working day. From this, nurses gain not only sympathy but also feedback on how they dealt with a particular situation.

Supervision is often negatively associated with more traditional disciplinary dealings between managers and their staff. These dealings are seen as punitive and can carry impressions born out of previous negotiations between superiors and novitiates, but this is a narrow definition and more generous interpretations are available. It has been suggested by Platt-Koch (1986) that the goals of supervision are to:

- expand the therapist's knowledge base;
- assist in developing clinical proficiency;
- develop autonomy and self-esteem as a professional.

These suggestions are ones with which the authors of this book would have considerable sympathy, indeed, a third contention of this book is that clinical supervision is an enabling process and involves not penalties but an opportunity for personal and professional growth. In her interesting review of the literature on supervision in the caring professions Hill (1980) examines the place of supervision in social work and clinical psychology and expresses surprise that supervision has not gained greater ground in nursing. Westheimer (1977) sees the supervisor in social work as ensuring scarce human and material resources are used to best advantage for the client, and identifies a role for supervisors in raising social work standards and in the allocation of case work. Hill (1989) makes the point that supervisors in social work appear to act as 'a buffer' between field social workers who provide client service and 'managers/policy makers'. A case could be made that nurses working in a health service with general management structures, need a similar provision of buffers.

An early substantive review of the literature and practice activity in various specialities by Butterworth and Faugier (1992) was one of the first to offer models for providing clinical supervision and mentorship for the health-care professions and to suggest mechanisms through which clinical supervision and mentorship could be drawn into practice.

Undoubtedly literature from other professions has affected the shaping of ideas about clinical supervision and mentorship in health care. Reported work in counselling and in psychotherapy provides useful models which have had considerable utility for mainstream health-care professionals (Hawkins and Shohet, 1989).The appropriateness of various theoretical models has had some debate and 'given truths' about existing ways of working are evident. Assertions that this is a 'counselling thing' or that clinical supervision is well-established in mental health care, or that 'midwives have been doing it for years' have been to some extent debunked as the wider implications of clinical supervision and mentorship have been recognized. Conversely, fears that this is a means of oversight and control by managers have largely dissipated, although, unfortunately, some employers use it in this way. A realization that the psychodynamic models often adopted by mental health professionals (Mahmood, 1994) or the organizational/structural models of midwifery (Harris, 1994) may be inappropriate for those working in acute surgery, intensive care or primary health care has dawned (Butterworth and Bishop, 1994) and the need to develop models which best serve the speciality and locality are necessary.

There appears to be an acceptance that the composite elements offered by Procter (1989) have found favour among the professions. Her description of the normative (organizational responsibility), formative (the development of skills) and restorative (supporting personal well-being) as the key elements of clinical supervision are popular, although some have taken issue with the terminology. The delivery of clinical supervision and mentorship often fashioned after ideas proposed by Houston (1990) has also started to shape up into 'ideal types'. One-to-one sessions with a supervisor from the same discipline have been reported (Dewing, 1994); one-to-one peer supervision has also been reported (Semperingham, 1994), but interestingly has been criticized as being the most likely method to be open to difficulty through the dangers of slipping into a consensus collusion (Faugier and Butterworth, 1994); peer group supervision has found favour particularly amongst district nurses and health visitors. While networking supervision is used in such specialist areas as HIV/AIDS care and Macmillan nursing, there appears to be no reported data. There has been a view that the cost consequences of implementing clinical supervision may hinder its implementation. However the little evidence that there is shows the consequences to be less significant than might be supposed (Dudley and Butterworth, 1994).

The international literature demonstrates some discussion in other countries on the subject. Inevitably because of socio-cultural differences, definitions have different meanings. However, some general observations are possible. Supervisors have a wide literature in the USA. The meaning is particular and refers most often to a 'superior/novitiate' type of relationship which has a strong management focus. The term 'clinical supervision' is sometimes used as a term of reference for supervisors, although the interpretation has no apparent difference. There have been more generous interpretations by authors seeking to develop the purpose of clinical supervision and mentorship to embrace personal and professional development although this type of discussion is less common.

There have been interesting debates around possible differences between mentorship and preceptorship (Darling, 1985). These sometimes have eye-catching titles such as 'What to do about toxic mentors' (op. cit.) and carry lessons of common interest to all those working in clinical supervision and mentorship. In Japan, nurses appear to have taken on USA models (Ito, 1984). German observers report a view which is more growth promoting and developmental (Olbrich, 1985) and Australians are beginning to raise the subject through conference agendas. Researchers in Scandinavia report some progress on action and evaluation of clinical supervision in mental health (Halberg and Norberg, 1993). There appears to be interest across the professions and while the debate is being raised in nursing as 'clinical supervision', in medicine it is being referred to as 'mentorship', and sometimes by health-care mangers as 'preceptorship'. Whatever the finer points of difference in the debate between them, the underpinning ideas are similar and the research findings reported have a common usefulness to all those who engage in clinical supervision and mentorship.

POLICY

Recommendations have been made about the importance of implementing clinical supervision both by the profession itself and the UK Department of Health. The Department of Health commissioned a review of the literature on clinical supervision and distributed it widely to the profession. In a letter which accompanied its distribution, (DoH, 1994) the Chief Nursing Officer said that:

'I have no doubt as to the value of clinical supervision and consider it to be fundamental to safeguarding standards, the development of professional expertise and the delivery of care'.

The King's Fund Centre has produced an account of five case studies from its nursing development units and suggested guidelines for introducing clinical supervision (Kohner, 1994). Recent reports and reviews on nursing, midwifery and health-visiting practice have given clinical supervision a central place in discussions and recommendations. This is most encouraging, and has raised the profile of clinical supervision so that clinicians, educators and researchers are giving the matter their attention.

However, clinical supervision *is not* and should *never be* 'yet another imposition from management or academics' placed on those in practice. Those with memories of having to 'do' the nursing process in a particular way or work within an ill-understood or inappropriate nursing theory, because a manager or educator was seized by the moment, will not take kindly to yet more of the same. Clinical supervision can both empower and support those in practice and must therefore be developed by and through them, as the process of clinical supervision rests on an immediate experience of clinical work and can only be realized by those actively working in practice.

The process of becoming a suitable supervisor is one which does not depend upon, nor is owned by a particular professional group. In a study by Brammer (1979), in which he looked at teachers, psychotherapists, priests and nurses, it is suggested that factors which allow users to recognize a 'good' person with which to form an interpersonal relationship do not depend upon a particular school of thought or ideological position. Rather, it is factors related to opportunity for intellectual and personal development which make the difference. These are clearly matters which would have an effect on an individual's potential as a mentor or supervisor.

Some working principles are offered here which are derived from the literature on clinical supervision.

SUPERVISION AS A PROTECTIVE DEVICE

It can be argued that supervision may provide a means of protection to nurses. Burnout and work-related stress often feature as causes for professional concern. The precipitant causes of burnout and stress are not yet clear. In a review of literature associated with stress, Copp (1988) suggests that stress can be viewed as both a stimulus and as a response and supports Cox's definition (1978) of stress as an imbalance between demand and coping where a stress response results when the individual fails to cope with a stimulus. Freudenburger's definition of burnout (1975) includes 'physical and emotional exhaustion involving the development of negative concepts, negative job attitudes and a loss of concern and feelings for clients'. McCarthy (1985) states:

'Nurses are particularly prone to burnout because of the lack of preparation for coping with emotional stress. They are seldom taught to specify their own needs, and they receive little or no training in interpersonal skills. It is not surprising therefore that many are unable to maintain their initial idealism, caring and commitment and the burnout process ensues.'

A variety of proposals have been offered which might make up a means of stress management. These include preventive measures involving relaxation and yoga and go on to providing more tertiary counselling services for nurses who are experiencing symptoms of burnout. The latter strategy would appear to be less useful, and it may be more important to strengthen nurses so that they can manage their work more comfortably. As Copp (1988) suggests in her summary, 'The ability to reduce stress through individual insight and self awareness may be the best method for nurses to lead more fulfilling lifestyles'. A system of clinical supervision in nursing may be the vehicle for providing this more rewarding way of working.

SOME DEFINITION OF TERMS

Having initially suggested that clinical supervision is an umbrella term for many things, it is becoming clear that it is possible to differentiate between clinical supervision, mentorship and the roles of assessor and preceptor. There is some danger in prescribing tight definitions to terminology when a field of knowledge is in an early period of growth. However there is some evidence of people wishing to combine the role of mentor and assessor (Northcott, 1989), a view which others might find incompatible. As the terms are therefore receiving some definitive attention by nursing, interpretation for the purposes of this book may help to clarify at least four of the terms which will occur repeatedly.

- Mentor – An experienced professional nurturing and guiding the novitiate, be they student or established professional.
- Assessor – An experienced professional making judgements on another's ability to carry out procedures or interactions.
- Clinical supervision – An exchange between practising professionals to enable the development of professional skills.
- Preceptor – A teacher or instructor.

ESTABLISHING GROUND RULES

Having visited the terminology, some positional statement is helpful, if only so that others might knock it down! In a profession which embraces mentorship and supervision it is permissable to identify a number of 'ground rules':

1 Skills should be constantly re-defined and improved throughout professional life.
2 Critical debate about practice activity is a means to professional development.
3 Clinical supervision offers protection to independent and accountable practice.
4 Introduction to a process of clinical supervision should begin in professional training and education, and continue thereafter as an integral part of professional development.
5 Clinical supervision requires time and energy and is not an incidental event.

These 'ground rules' can be further expanded.

1. Skills should be constantly re-defined and improved throughout professional life

It is not difficult to accept that, once nurses have qualified, their skills will continue to develop as more experiences are met and worked through. Current thoughts on post-qualifying professional development in nursing would support this, and it is clear that a learning curve continues for some years after qualification. There must be a point, however, where new experiences are less common and a plateau in learning is reached. Ten years of clinical experience might well consist of two years of new experiences and personal development followed by eight years in which there are no new challenges needing different solutions. It is possible, therefore, that stagnation and complacency might emerge where no ongoing attention is given to developing skills in qualified staff.

2. Critical debate about practice activity is a means to professional development

There are limited opportunities for nurses to engage in critical debate about practice activities. Nurses are not expected to set aside time specifically to consider how best to nurse a patient and his/her family. Case conferences for nurses are a rare event and yet common enough in the preparation and education of students. Even within a multi-disciplinary setting contributions from nurses are often limited. An example, although somewhat exaggerated, serves to make the point. In a ward round medical staff will often agonize over the finer points of diagnosis, social workers will deliver an analysis of social circumstances, psychologists give a list of mental tests, occupational therapists explicate a range of rehabilitative programmes. When asked (if asked!) the nurse might contribute by saying 'slept well' or 'up and about' or 'moved bowels'. Offerings are limited because nurses are not practised in putting forward a contribution which will stand up to critical review and grows from a belief that to be criticized means that your ideas must be wrong. This, in turn, is a self-inflicted injury brought about by a process of education which has not used critical analysis of practice and believes that there is always a 'right answer'.

Because nurses do not often indulge in critical debate as a matter of routine, they are not expected to make a significant contribution to case conferences. Exposure to case conferences is part of a process of clinical supervision and can help to develop those skills central to an ability to participate in critical debate related to practice.

3. Clinical supervision offers protection to independent and accountable practice

In recent times, a bid for independent and accountable practice has grown in nursing. This bid has manifested itself in a call for advanced nurse practitioners and assertions that nurses are responsible and, therefore, accountable for their own practice. It is not yet clear if nursing is professionally equipped to handle the consequences of independence and responsibility.

Stillwell (1988) has suggested that nurse practitioners need to be sure that:

- a nurse can practise safely when patients have open access to their extended skills;
- an extended/expanded role is acceptable to patients;
- an extended/expanded role is acceptable to colleagues.

Advanced practice depends upon proper preparation through education and skill development. The advanced nurse will need a safe professional framework in which to practise – what has been called 'protected autonomy'. This can only be achieved by introducing the concept of clinical supervision into the profession as a whole, not just to enable the development of the nurse practitioner role but beginning at first level nurse training and continuing through to the nurse consultant. The rise of a litigation-minded public and less than total defence of assumed vicarious liability by employers brings an added complication to developing the role of the nurse practitioner. Responsibility for action and, more importantly extended action must become part and parcel of nursing's 'professional baggage'. Nurses have a strong professional voice through the Royal College of Nursing and they have made their position clear. Two of their documents, *Boundaries of Nursing* (RCN, 1988a) and *Specialities in Nursing* (RCN, 1988b) make the case. The first of these two publications, *Boundaries in Nursing*, suggests:

'The boundaries of nursing must be able to respond to people's needs. Educational curricula and official guidelines however tend to change relatively slowly. It is nurses themselves who are faced with making the decisions as to what they will, and will not do, since each nurse is accountable for his or her professional practice.'

Clearly there is room for professional growth within these boundaries. The second, *Specialities in Nursing*, makes the case with greater force:

'If the profession of nursing is to reach its ultimate goal of providing relevant nursing care to meet individual patient's needs, then ultimately the role of the nurse specialist is central to its achievement.'

This claim builds on propositions earlier in the document that nurse specialists are:

'experts in a particular aspect of nursing care – they demonstrate refined clinical practice, either as a result of significant experience or advanced expertise, or a knowledge in a branch or speciality'.

These are obvious requirements for advanced practice and the profession has laid a claim which determines two steps leading to its realization: expert knowledge or clinical skill and permission to break the boundaries of previously defined roles.

4. Introduction to a process of clinical supervision should begin in professional training and education, and continue thereafter as an integral part of professional development

At the introduction of the Nurses, Midwives and Health Visitors Act in 1979, some debate was raised about the requirement for the maintenance of a 'live' register. In order to stay on the UKCC register, qualified nurses and health visitors have to pay a periodic re-registration fee. However, with the exception of midwives, no requirement to demonstrate competence is required in order to stay on the register. It has now been argued that some mandatory in-service education should be provided in order that those on the register are aware of research and changes in practice, thus giving the register a membership of up-to-date practitioners (UKCC, 1990). There has been little debate on how to test the clinical skills of those on the register, and it could be argued that clinical supervision might provide some confidence in the clinical competence of those on the register.

The UKCC has produced statements both on recommendations for a period of preceptorship (UKCC, 1995) and on clinical supervision (UKCC, 1996). They suggest that although neither needs statutory requirement, certain matters of principle and good practice should obtain.

5. Clinical supervision requires time and energy and is not an incidental event

The British Association for Counselling have made recommendations that their recognized supervisors will have 'an on-going arrangement for consultation and supervision'. This implies that there is a specific time commitment to clinical supervision and that those doing it are available and in practice. It is evident that those carrying out clinical supervision in nursing will need to be familiar with, and expert in, clinical practice. There are some so-called 'clinical manager' positions which are held by nurses who have not practised for a considerable period and their ability to give clinical supervision must be questionable. Happily, this is not generally the case and the level of clinical expertise available is often of the highest quality.

It will take time to absorb the principles of clinical supervision into nursing and its day-to-day activities. However, it appears fashionable to not move forward on anything unless it can somehow be tied to patient-led outcomes and evidence-based practice, as though these laudable aims were achievable overnight! This is an objective to which we must all strive, but more often complex matters such as these will take considerable time to achieve and we must not reject non-evidence-based practice as being either wrong or necessarily of poor quality. A sure sign of success for clinical supervision will be when it has become part of the cultural 'norm' for nurses, midwives and health visitors and does not require the special attention that it now gets in order to implement it in the clinical setting. A future dream is to see any absence of clinical supervision as a curiosity, and when this is so we can be sure that its enculteration into the professions is complete.

REFERENCES

Brammer, L. (1979) *The Helping Relationship*. Prentice-Hall, New York.

Burnard, P. (1988) Mentors: A supporting act, *Nursing Times*, 16 Nov., **84**(66).

Burnard, P. (1989) The role of mentor, *Journal of District Nursing*, **8**(3), 8–17.

Butterworth, C. A. (1988) *Breaking the Boundaries; New Endeavours in Community Nursing*, Inaugural Lecture, University of Manchester.

Butterworth, C. A. (1990) *The Nurse Practitioner in the United Kingdom*, Paper given to the National Organization of Nurse Practitioner Faculty, University of Texas, Galveston.

Butterworth, T. and Bishop, V. (eds) (1994) *Clinical Supervision: A Report of the Trust Nurse Executive Workshops*, NHS Executive/HMSO, London.

Butterworth, T. and Faugier, J. (1992) *Clinical Supervision and Mentorship in Nursing*, Stanley Thornes, Cheltenham.

Copp, G. (1988) The reality behind stress, *Nursing Times*, 9 Nov., **84**(45).

Cox, T. (1978) *Stress*, Macmillan, New York.

Darling, L. A. (1984) What do nurses want in a mentor? *Journal of Nursing Administration*, Oct., **14**(10),42–4.

Darling, L. A. (1985) What to do about toxic mentors, *Journal of Nursing Administration*, May, **15**(5) 43–4.

DoH (1994) CNO Letter 94(5) Clinical supervision for the nursing and health visiting professions.

Dewing, J. (1994) *Report on Burford Community Hospital*, in Kohner, N. (ed.) (1994) op. cit.

Dudley, M. and Butterworth, T. (1994) The costs and some benefits of clinical supervision: An initial exploration, *The International Journal of Psychiatric Nursing Research*, **1**(2), 34–40.

English National Board (ENB) (1994) *Study of the Relationships Between Teaching, Support, Supervision and Role Modelling for Students in Clinical Areas in the Context of Project 2000 Courses*, ENB, London.

English National Board for Nurses, Midwives and Health Visitors (ENB) (1989) *Preparation of Teachers, Practitioner/Teachers, Mentors and Supervisors in the Context of Project 2000*, ENB, London.

Faugier, J. and Butterworth, T. (1994) *Clinical Supervision: A Position Paper*, School of Nursing Studies, The University of Manchester, UK.

Freudenberger, H. J. (1975) The staff burn-out syndrome, *Psychotherapy: Theory, Research and Practice*, **12**, 73–82.

Goldberg, D. and Williams, P. (1988) *A User's Guide to the General Health Questionnaire*, NFER-Nelson, Windsor, UK.

Halberg, I. R. and Norberg, A. (1993) Strain among nurses and their emotional reactions during one year of systematic clinical supervision combined with the implementation of individualized care in dementia nursing, *Journal of Advanced Nursing*, **18**, 1860–75.

Harris, L. (1994) Report on midwifery supervision in South Thames Regional Health Authority, in Butterworth, T. and Bishop, V. (eds) (1994) op. cit.

Hawkins, P. and Shohet, R. (1989) *Supervision in the Helping Professions*, Open University Press, Milton Keynes, UK.

Hill, J. (1989) Supervision in the caring professions: A literature review, *Community Psychiatric Nursing Journal*, Oct., **9**(5), 9–15.

Houston, G. (1990) *Supervision and Counselling*, The Rochester Foundation, London.

Ito, S. (1984) *Kangogaku Zasshi*, Dec., **48**(12), 1405.

Jarvis, P. and Gibson S. (1985) *The Teacher Practitioner in Nursing, Midwifery and Health Visiting*, Croom Helm, London.

Kohner, N. (ed.) (1994) *Clinical Supervision in Practice*, King's Fund Centre, London/BEBC, Dorset, UK.

Mahmood, N (1994) Report on Cartmel Ward Prestwich Hospital, in Kohner, N. (ed.) (1994) op. cit.

McCarthy, P. (1985) Burnout in psychiatric nursing, *Journal of Advanced Nursing*, **10**, 305–10.

Menzies, I. E. P. (1960) *The Functioning of Social Systems as a Defense Against*

Anxiety: A Report on a Study of the Nursing Service of a General Hospital, Tavistock, London.

Northcott, N. (1989) Mentorship in nurse education, *Nursing Standard*, 11 March, **13**(24), 25.

Olbrich, C. (1985) Supervision as a possibility for nursing personal to reflect on professional behaviour and expand professional competence, *Krankenpfledge*, **39**(5), 181–3.

Pearson, A. (1988) *Primary Nursing: Nursing in the Burford and Oxford Nursing Development Units*, Croom Helm, London.

Platt-Koch, L. M. (1986) Clinical supervision for psychiatric nurses, *Journal of Psycho-Social Nursing*, **26**(1), 7–15.

Procter, B. (1989) On being a trainer: Training and supervision for counselling in action, in Hawkins, B. and Shohet, R. (eds) (1989) op. cit.

Puetz, B.E. (1985) Learn the ropes from a mentor, *Nursing Success Today*, **2**(6), 11–13.

Rogers, C. (1951) *Client Centred Therapy*, Constable, London.

RCN (1988a) *Specialties in Nursing: A Report of the Working Party Investigating the Development of Specialties within the Nursing Profession*, RCN, London.

RCN (1988b) *Boundaries of Nursing: A Policy Statement*, RCN, London.

Semperingham, J. (1994) Report on Eillen Skellern Three Ward, in Kohner, N. (ed.) (1994) op. cit.

Spouse, J. (1996) The effective mentor: A model for student-centred learning in clinical practice, *NT Research*, **1**(2), 120–33.

Stilwell, B. (1988) Patient attitudes to a highly developed extended role: The nurse practitioner, *Recent Advances in Nursing*, **21**, 82–100.

Stockwell, E. (1972) *The Unpopular Patient*, RCN, London.

UKCC (1990) *The Report of the Post-Registration Education and Practice Project, (PREPP)*, UKCC, London.

UKCC (1995) The Council's position concerning a period of support and preceptorship: Implementation of the post-registration education and practice project. Registrar's letter 4 January 1993, UKCC, London.

UKCC (1996) *Position Statement on Clinical Supervision for Nursing and Health Visiting*, UKCC, London.

Weiss, D., Dawis, R., England, G. and Lofquist, L. (1967) Manual for the Minnesota Satisfaction Questionnaire. University of Minnesota Industrial Relations Centre, Minnesota.

Westheimer, I. J. (1977) *The Practice of Supervision in Social Work*, Ward Lock Educational, London.

White, E. (1996) Clinical supervision and Project 2000: The identification of some substantive issues, *NT Research*, **1**(2), 102–11.

Wright, S. G. (1986) *Building and Using a Model of Nursing*, Edward Arnold, London.

The supervisory relationship

Jean Faugier

In striving to improve their understanding and practice of nursing, nurses have recognized the importance of a supervisory relationship which is outside traditional hierarchical roles. The term 'supervision' conjures up for nurses ideas of discipline and criticism, and for many of them it is a word with more managerial than clinical connotations. Watts (1987) suggests that:

> 'The generally held conception of supervision is of a lower management activity in which a group of workers is overseen by a supervisor for a variety of reasons such as ensuring timekeeping, processing pay entitlements, regulating rates of work, and monitoring the quality of work according to pre-set standards.'

That nurses at all levels, from senior nursing staff to students, require a relationship which focuses primarily on the process and experience of nursing, is something which the profession has been slow to accept. There are of course notable examples of the opposite, both nationally and internationally: nurses in North America have for some time now adopted a more psychodynamic/humanist understanding of the individual and many general and psychiatric nurses in the United States have established supervisory and mentor relationships which focus on these philosophies. In the UK, pockets of psychiatric and general nurses working in specialized or community settings have for some time been acutely aware of the importance of clinical supervision in improving their skills. Barber and Norman (1987) describe supervision as:

> 'an interpersonal process in which the skilled practitioner helps a less skilled or experienced practitioner to achieve professional abilities appropriate to his role, at the same time being offered counsel and support.'

In order to develop these relationships, which were previously not thought to be essential to good nursing practice, nurses have been forced to adopt models from other disciplines. Whilst there is indeed a wealth of experience and some excellent texts on supervision in areas such as social work, psychotherapy and teaching, it is often only through the adoption of a new philosophical orientation that nurses can obtain experience of these models. Although the impetus for the development of whatever supervision exists within nursing has undoubtedly come from those nurses who have taken that step, it is neither possible nor desirable for all nurses to shift their philosophical orientation from nursing to psychotherapeutic, social or educational models.

In skilled hands, however, such theoretical and practical experience from other disciplines can have a very beneficial effect. The skilled nurse with experience of supervision in psychotherapy, for example, should be capable of selectively adapting psychodynamic supervision for use in nursing situations. Unfortunately, all too often such models are transferred lock, stock and barrel, and as such are experienced as inappropriate and limited, with little reference to the nurse's role.

In those areas where nurses have managed to develop models of excellence in supervision of clinical practice, they may be viewed by colleagues as elitist and removed from the real experience of the 'average nurse'. Nursing has traditionally been intolerant and suspicious of anything which smacks of indulgence, and it can effectively deal with fears of such developments by isolating those practitioners, labelling them as different from the mainstream. As Ivey (1977) writes:

'Supervision in the helping profession has too long been considered an art form reserved only for the master practitioner.'

In the course of this chapter, we hope to provide guidelines to good practice in developing and managing the supervisory relationship in nursing settings.

It behoves us first to examine the nature of the supervisory relationship described by writers from related professions. Without this, we are in danger of re-inventing the wheel, and possibly a wheel of inferior quality.

Almost echoing the developments in nursing in the last few years, Westheimer (1977) bemoaned the lack of importance attributed to supervision in social work:

'There is much general ignorance about the nature and process of supervision, with its major objective of bringing about an effective client service. Social workers who find themselves promoted overnight to the position of supervisor receive little help, if any, with their new functions and tasks. Mostly they are not secure enough to declare their needs for further education in this sphere, afraid of being thought incompetent.'

Since the post-Seebohm (1968) days in which Westheimer was writing, further reorganizations of social work have served to underline the importance of the supervisor's role and the need for its further development. The arrival of scores of newly-trained social workers in inner-city areas with inadequate levels of casework supervision continues to be a grave cause for concern to the profession and society, often only being revealed in a somewhat dramatic manner when a case goes tragically wrong for the want of experienced input to case supervision. However, some outstanding work on supervision has been achieved in the field of social work by such theorists as Kadushin (1976) and Pettes (1979) whose pioneering efforts have done much to make casework supervision an accepted and expected part of practice for social workers of all grades.

The other major contribution to our understanding of the nature of supervisory practice has come from psychotherapy. Drawing largely on the experience of clinical supervision as undertaken in psychoanalysis, the major emphasis here is a study of the interactive and communications systems contained in the therapist–client relationship and the therapist–supervisor relationship. This form of clinical supervision is often very structured and involves a complicated network of motivations revealed in the triadic dimensions of the supervisory relationship. Inevitably, a treatment orientation such as psychoanalysis, which concentrates on working with the unconscious life of the patient, will essentially reflect such an orientation in the supervisory process. Long-term treatment of patients over many years is mirrored by similar long term relationships between supervisors and supervisees, in which the defences and resistances of the trainee therapist are as interesting to the supervisor as those of the patient, and often more so, as they frequently represent evidence of transference relationships developing in the therapeutic process. Wolberg (1988) writes:

'It is almost inevitable that psychotherapists will be influenced by unconscious processes in their patients. Patients who have incorporated parental messages and repudiated their presence may through projective identification accuse the therapist of the very impulses which they deny in themselves. More insidiously, the projections may not be direct, but the therapist will become aware of them through countertransference, perhaps reflected in dreams or fantasies.'

The understanding of these processes is absolutely vital to the safe practice of psychotherapy, and writers such as Langs (1979) point out that a failure to recognize such phenomena through the medium of supervision can lead to destructive acting out behaviour by the therapist, typified by feelings of aggression or smothering overprotectiveness. One of the prime duties of the supervisor is to assist the supervisee to recognize such communications when they occur and to work through them via the medium of the supervisory relationship rather than the therapeutic one. This model of supervisory practice works within strict contractual boundaries over lengthy periods of training, and whilst such intensive supervision is highly desirable for those wishing to work as psychotherapists, it is not appropriate for those who have shorter-term, less intensive, therapeutic relationships. Analysts such as Balint (1957), Malan (1975) and Hobson (1985) have clearly recognized this shortcoming and have adapted psychodynamic models to shorter-term therapeutic work.

These models which, just like all psychodynamic work, are based on the requirement of good quality supervision, have been used successfully with general practitioners, nurses and social workers in particular.

THE SUPERVISORY RELATIONSHIP IN PSYCHOTHERAPY

Describing the manner in which various influences have shaped the view of supervision in psychotherapy, Wolberg (1988) claims that skilled supervisors must deftly weave their way through the sometimes very disparate needs of the supervisees, patients and institutions, until they can somehow fuse the various elements into a serviceable amalgam. Whilst not discounting the earlier influences of psychoanalysis, supervision in psychotherapy is currently moving towards a more eclectic model in which the primary function is not 'therapy' for the supervisee, but concentrates instead on the educational and evaluative elements of the supervisory situation.

Increasingly, supervision is being viewed as an essential educational process, vital to the acquisition of effective therapeutic skills, and central to professional growth. Supervision is about the overall functioning of the therapist in the clinical situation, and this is unlikely to be assessed by concentrating solely on the unconscious of the trainee. It is, however, unlikely to be assessed fully should this be ignored. In order to achieve this balance in therapeutic practice, it may be necessary to bring to the supervisees' attention the fact that they have failed to live up to therapeutic potential, either due to lack of knowledge or skill, or because of unresolved neurotic character traits which impinge on the relationship with patient or supervisor.

When identifying personal problems in the supervisee, it is not the role of the supervisor to change the emphasis from supervision to therapy, but to raise awareness in the hope that the supervisee will be encouraged to undertake personal therapy to resolve such issues. The primary task of supervision is to assist supervisees to gain knowledge that is lacking, to help them to establish and maintain the therapeutic relationship, to overcome resistances to learning, and to undertake an evaluation of their skills and capacities for the purpose of professional development. By providing a 'safe environment', the supervisor in psychotherapy can help the supervisee to make great strides in theoretical understanding, therapeutic aptitudes, and abilities to form and sustain relationships with both patients and supervisors.

THE SUPERVISORY RELATIONSHIP IN SOCIAL WORK

In attempting to prioritize the requirements of the supervisor's role in social work practice, Westheimer (1977) places the emphasis on the educational elements:

> 'Supervision is an individual method of learning further in the performance of a responsible job. To help people learn, to ask questions in a way which leads to well considered and appropriate decision, calls for theoretical knowledge, practical skills, and experience as a competent social worker.'

Westheimer goes on to attempt to delineate the requirements of the supervisor in furthering knowledge: the possession and consolidation of knowledge, teaching skill, empathy for clients and colleagues, enjoyment in the development of others, familiarity with agency structure, an ability to regulate emotional pressures, appropriate use of authority, and a willingness to develop. Clearly supervision is not a task for those lacking in either experience or insight.

Also examining the functions of the supervisory role, Middleman and Rhodes (1985) point out that the most frequently expressed desire of workers in the field, as is so often the case in nursing, relates to the areas of increased autonomy and esteem in respect of their individual practice. In an attempt to facilitate such developments, they postulate nine areas of emphasis for the would-be social work supervisor:

1. the personal and interpersonal aspects of supervision;
2. encouraging self acceptance;
3. giving feedback;
4. encouraging interpersonal regard, the development of trust, caring and interdependence;
5. managing tension;
6. helping the supervisee deal with uncertainties, and fostering clinical autonomy;
7. facilitating the recognition of clinical boundaries and limitations in skill and competence;
8. enhancing morale in order to inspire and motivate towards excellence;
9. helping supervisees recognize the service delivery functions of their role, in order to respond to the client in conformity with the ethical bases and values of the profession.

LESSONS FOR NURSING

There can be little doubt that a close examination of the functions of the supervisor and the nature of the supervisory relationship would prove useful to nursing. However, the rather piecemeal nature of its development has resulted in a fragmented understanding within the nursing profession of the importance of supervision in clinical practice. Frequently, one sees 'the need for supervision' tacked on to the end of a training programme or a description of a nursing model as if it is something which simply happens. It would seem that our colleagues from social work and psychotherapy have learned some time ago that unless a thorough examination of what is meant by clinical supervision is undertaken, time set aside for it to happen, and an outline of the duties and requirements of the supervisor clearly made, it is likely to remain an unfulfilled demand repeated at every opportunity by clinical workers.

In the past decade, much has been written about the need for supervision in nursing, but comparatively little has been written on effective techniques, or on the roles and requirements within the supervisory relationship. Recently there have been exciting developments in the profession which have involved the integration of previously discrete clinical orientations. Behaviourists are now seen in open dialogue with psychodynamic colleagues, counselling co-exists alongside 'high-tech' approaches, such as invasive surgery and investigation; the influence of complementary therapies on the practice of a great many nurses is now an established fact. Supervision of such diverse clinical practice must itself take an eclectic framework if it is to contain the all important elements of education and support whilst resisting the temptation to become too rigid and dogmatic. The need pragmatically to blend clinical models is common even in areas of clinical practice which claim a strong adherence to one philosophical position. Day-to-day experience with patients and clients underlines the need for such flexibility, if we are to avoid imposing our 'favourite' approach to treatment and care upon them inappropriately.

A similar approach has been developed by Halgin (1986) to the supervisory relationship:

'The realm of individual supervision is an optimal format within which to communicate to trainees the excitement of the growing trend to therapeutic integration. Not only can teachers convey to supervisees the utility of therapeutic integration, but they have the invaluable opportunity to demonstrate it to them within the context of the supervisory relationship.'

Just as one would expect the nurse to have the ability selectively to blend various clinical approaches in response to the patients' needs, the supervisor should be able to demonstrate such an ability during clinical supervision. Examples from psychodynamic theory, behavioural theory, interpersonal humanistic theories, biological theories and sociological theories all have a major contribution to make to a working model of clinical supervision for nurses.

THE GROWTH AND SUPPORT MODEL OF THE SUPERVISORY RELATIONSHIP

In an attempt to provide some guidelines to the characteristics of the supervisory relationship which are essential to good practice, we offer here one particular way of looking at the various elements.

The role of the supervisor is to facilitate *growth* both educationally and personally in the supervisee, whilst providing essential *support* to their developing clinical autonomy. In order to achieve this, the supervisor must be aware of elements of the relationship for which they are responsible.

Generosity

This is an essential requirement in a supervisor or mentor, and does not simply refer to supplying the coffee during the supervision session, although the provision of such seemingly unimportant items can add significantly to the atmosphere and experience of supervision. In particular, supervisors will need to be generous with their time, which is often precious and in short supply, especially to the experienced trained nurse responsible for the well-being of patients as well as colleagues. Instructions such as: 'Let's see if we can find some time tomorrow, shall we?', or 'Make sure you bring that issue up when I am on duty next' can be extremely discouraging to supervisees who may fear that they will be considered pestering and inadequate if they request supervision.

This inability to place clinical supervision in a position of priority means that all other activities, such as answering the telephone, dealing with enquiries and with medical staff, attending to administration, etc., are always eating into the time needed for supervision.

It is also important that the supervisor displays a generosity of spirit. Supervision with someone who finds it difficult to give either intellectually or emotionally within the supervisory relationship will be unsuccessful in providing the all important inspiration which can only arise truly from a well-managed transference relationship. Significantly too, supervision with an absence of generosity can be a very punitive experience, leaving the supervisee confused and angry.

Rewarding

Development and effort deserve to be rewarded. A supervisee will frequently display marked ability in certain areas at an exceptionally high level. It is the duty of the mature supervisor (the term is used with no reference to age, but implies that the supervisor has been through the processes now being experienced by the supervisee, and has derived some insight from the journey) to further such development by rewarding in the form of praise and encouragement. It is not appropriate for any supervisor or mentor to use the supervisory relationship to deal with unresolved feelings of inadequacy or insecurity. Self awareness is therefore a prerequisite for selection as a supervisor and the institution or service should ensure that such training is undertaken prior to working in a responsible position as a supervisor. Moreover, such self-awareness should of course be ongoing, and supervisors themselves should have access to either personal or group supervision in order to facilitate this process. Casement (1985) emphasizes this process of self-development contained within the supervisor's role:

'Just as we can see our own errors more clearly in others, so too in supervising others. Here there are endless opportunities for therapists to re-examine their own work, when looking closely at the work of the person being supervised. Not infrequently, supervisors will be seeing reflections of their own difficulties with technique. We do not always do as we teach others to do, but we can learn a lot by trying.'

Although writing about psychotherapy, Bion (1975) coined the term which perhaps exemplifies this process of continued self-awareness development necessary in the supervisor, when he claimed we should always be in a state of becoming. Those nurses who, upon qualifying, feel that they know all they need to know, not only about nursing but also about themselves, should never be given the opportunity to stunt the growth of others through the medium of supervision.

Openness

In the course of supervising a process as complex and demanding as nursing, difficult and awkward times will frequently occur. The real nature of our human existence, characterized by uncertainty, tension, confusion, irritation, and anger, is vividly displayed when illness occurs, either in ourselves or those we care for. The problems which nurses have in coping with this tapestry of emotional and physical responses can and is often mirrored in the supervisory process. Problems and tensions which arise between supervisor and supervisee can, in effect, often turn out to be the very essence of the learning experience, allowing the supervisee to give voice to something which would otherwise remain a worrying feeling. The authors have frequently been in the position of 'not knowing' in the supervision of others. This is particularly true when the material presented for supervision is very distressing or disturbing, or the physical condition of the patient is life threatening, disabling or disfiguring.

The tradition in nursing is for the person in the educational role such as the clinical supervisor to provide the answers, to be all knowing. And yet the most important learning experience the supervisor can provide is openness to feelings and experience, i.e. simply being able to stay with the feelings of the supervisee and therefore vicariously with the patient. The need to fill voids and cover gaps by intervention has always been nursing's way of dealing with anxiety, and it is important for the supervisor not to become an example of this.

The *parallel process*, identified by Ekstein and Wallenstein (1958), refers to the analogy between the experience of the patient–supervisee relationship and that of the supervisor–supervisee. For example, a nurse who is angry with the world and medical science for failing to help a young male patient dying with HIV, angry with the young man himself for leaving her when she is now so fond of him, and angry with herself for also not being able to be the 'perfect nurse' who would avoid such feelings, will almost certainly express some of these feelings at some stage in supervision in the form of overt or covert anger and hostility towards the supervisor whom she perhaps perceives as failing to keep her protected from these painful emotions. It is in these difficult times that much of the real learning about nursing will take place, by supervisors displaying an ability to remain open to such parallel processes and using them to gain a greater understanding of all concerned, including themselves. At times like this, when feelings are on the surface, it will help the supervisor to remember the old maxim that 'anyone can hold the helm when the sea is calm'.

Willingness to learn

Nursing organization, infested as it is with the constraints of hierarchy, can appear to be a system loaded against the development of continued learning. Sensitivity to position and seniority are handicaps which hamper the recognition of personal limitations and the ability to listen to others. This threat of losing position or 'face' before junior or untrained members of staff arises from a serious misconception endemic in nursing: the belief that one can ever know all there is to know even about one's own role and that such knowledge is static. As George Bernard Shaw pointed out in *Major Barbara*: 'You have learned something, that always feels as though you have lost something.' How many of us have felt that gradual loss of certainty in our careers as we have moved from the completion of training, to face the ambiguity at the heart of our profession?

Supervisors who fail to maintain an ability to continue learning throughout their careers are denying the very dynamic nature of nursing, and will be in constant fear of being engulfed by the oncoming tide of development represented by the person of their supervisees.

Thoughtful and thought-provoking

The participants in the supervisory process invariably bring to the situation their own agenda. The supervisees are interested in learning 'nursing' or some special related skill, in order to gain a qualification or obtain promotion. The supervisor, on the other hand, wishes to demonstrate competence as a senior clinical nurse whilst providing an environment in which supervisees can safely grow in terms of skill and intellect. The hospital, institution or service wishes to ensure that the patient receives a certain standard of nursing care, and sees supervision as one way of ensuring this. The many and various aims and aspirations placed upon the supervisory process can have the effect of diverting it from one of its two major roles, the *educative function*. The provision of adequate learning for supervisees presupposes an ability to present material in a way which will enable them to make the necessary cognitive links. Wolberg (1988) uses a particularly vivid example to draw attention to this need to stimulate intellectual understanding in supervisees:

> 'A professional coach who sends his or her players out to complete a number of practice games, with instructions on what to do, and who asks them to provide a verbal report at intervals of how they played and what they intended to do next, would probably last no more than one season. What is lacking is a systematic critique of actual performances as observed by peers and supervisors.'

The 'coach', then, must lead from the front, must have access to actual data in the form of observations, recordings or video material, and must seek to stimulate thought by offering informed theory-based links to the practice problems of the supervisee. All this of course demands a knowledge base on the part of the supervisor.

Humanity

McFarlane (1982) described nursing as the *art of caring*. By its very nature, nursing is a profession touched by the sorrows and joys of humankind in a very special way. The privileged position of being the person who provides intimate physical care to people in their times of greatest need and dependence is the basis of all good nursing. In order to fulfil our function to a high standard and retain the inherent dignity of those for whom we care, we must have within ourselves, and instil in those we supervise, a sense of that dignity. Supervisors will reflect this by the way they set the tone for the discussion of patients and their problems, and accept human frailties.

Humour is not out of place in supervision however; human beings are frequently comical characters. Perhaps the best example of supervisors' humanity is their ability to treat supervisees as worthy human beings in whose development they are privileged to be involved.

Sensitivity

A supervision session is a live encounter in the 'here and now' between two human beings. It is inevitable that each person brings to that encounter their uniqueness as an individual. It is also inevitable that each of the participants brings with them issues which are currently important for them outside of that situation. Sensitivity to personal and interpersonal work barriers is a crucial feature of effective supervision. Nursing has traditionally been a hierarchical and organizationally bureaucratic profession, noted for its tendency to over-emphasize the technical and organizational at the expense of the personal and interpersonal. A clear reflection of this tendency is seen in the reinforcing and rewarding of impersonality in relationships, defined as 'professionalism', the emphasis in nursing on behavioural strategies as 'separate problems', and the compartmentalization of task allocation. Such an approach results in a corresponding lack of concern for the whole person; it also works against the development of confident nurses with high personal regard for themselves and others. A feeling that one is appreciated, needed, and a sense that one's work is progressing along valued lines, are all essential aspects of producing self-acceptance in nursing. Frequently a supervisee will bring to supervision what they believe sincerely to be their best effort. Sometimes this best effort will have failed to produce anything but a disappointing outcome, or else an intervention will be viewed too optimistically by the supervisee. Middleman and Rhodes (1985) point out that, in such circumstances, it is too easy to give blanket common-sense responses to the frustrations and disappointments of the supervisee, when what is needed are 'uncommon-sense' responses: as a supervisor, it is necessary to give a response which reflects a sensitive appreciation of the work which has been put in, and the subsequent feelings of failure and guilt when the supervisee realizes that much of the effort may have been misguided, or has failed to show the hoped for results. This ability to value the nurse and her efforts can lead to the supervision session being used effectively for the purpose of education, i.e. exploring all the alternative strategies and interventions possible in the examined clinical situation.

Uncompromising

The dictionary definition of 'uncompromising' is 'not allowing or seeking compromise', 'unyielding or stubborn'. At first glance, this hardly seems a feature one would wish to include in a 'progressive' model of nursing supervision. And yet an uncompromising rigour is one of the most vital contributions an effective supervisor can bring to the overall process. The practice of nursing cannot be open to any compromise in the standards of care for individual patients, and this should be reflected in the supervisory process: by making use of probing casework, peer group assessment, supervisor observation, and the interpretation of individual presentations, the supervisor can maintain an atmosphere in which warmth and understanding go hand-in-hand with clinical and intellectual rigour. In addition, supervisors must establish an atmosphere of uncompromising confidentiality, trust, and professionalism. These issues, particularly that of the maintenance of therapeutic boundaries, can be demonstrated to the supervisee as part of the relationship within supervision, which may then be applied to other relationships outside, with patients and staff in the clinical setting.

The most difficult task of supervision is often the acknowledgement of problems 'seated' in oneself, and the need for more awareness of such issues. Supervisees sometimes employ classic 'approach avoidance' mechanisms in order to deal with such difficulties, and an uncompromising rigour is once again needed to ensure that supervisees make the necessary links not only with theory and practice, but also with their own feelings.

Personal

Supervision of clinical practice may be carried out in a great number of settings and styles. It will nevertheless have some essentially common features: it should, by definition, centre on the clinical work of nursing, the central focus of which is the relationship – the vehicle of nursing; additionally, it will commonly have an educational function and should therefore seek to increase self-awareness on the part of the supervisee.

Despite these common elements, however, it remains a personal experience, and should not be subjected to any unnecessary structure. Each individual supervisor or mentor will display an individual personal style, and it is important to consider and give due merit to this individuality when asking nurses to choose a supervisor. Sadly, the move to mentorship and clinical supervision in nursing has been marked in too many cases by a lack of understanding of the personal nature of the supervisory relationship, which has only contributed to devaluing the process and reducing its effectiveness in improving practice. The all-pervading notion that 'any nurse can nurse any patient' is transposed lock stock and barrel to supervision and becomes 'any supervisor can supervise any supervisee'. This is patently not the case, and simply serves to perpetuate the celebration of the impersonal which runs throughout our development as a profession.

Practical

Any supervision session in which a nurse does not acquire new skills in delivery of care, even if she feels more self-aware, constitutes a failure. Nursing is a practically-based profession. Care is delivered not only through emotional regard and psychological input, but also by the very practical measures which are vital to the patients' well being as well as representing a tangible expression of care. The educational process of supervision must therefore focus on practice and its improvement.

The development of *knowledge*, *attitudes*, and *skills* in nursing often places too little emphasis on the latter. In a profession that for decades has been plagued by a pragmatic approach to the 'how' of practice with little regard for the 'what' and the 'why', we have recently, and somewhat self-consciously, reversed the coin in an attempt to understand theoretical and attitudinal issues in greater depth. Whilst this is extremely important, it carries with it the danger of ignoring the practical issues of the 'how', with the result that clinical practice can, and does, suffer. The effective supervisor must guard against an over-intellectual, woolly approach to essentially practical interventions; neither must he/she assume that the supervisee will intuitively know 'how' to do 'what'. Clinical supervisors in nursing are provided with a wonderful opportunity in providing 'skills modelling' training. An example of this is provided by Brammer and Wassmer (1979) in their description of supervising trainee counsellors. In pointing to the dearth of outcome measures in counselling training, they plead the case for more focus on the 'behaviours' of supervisees as well as on knowledge and attitudes.

Orientation

As Wolberg (1988) points out, important and often irreconcilable differences occur in the theoretical background and orientation of the supervisor and the supervisee. Such differences may express themselves in nursing in any of the following ways:

1. the relative weight placed on biological as opposed to psychological and social factors in the genesis of a patient's problems;
2. the value of particular forms of intervention, particularly when such intervention may be seen as invasive and distressing for the patient;
3. the degree of stress which is placed on personality or character issues in determining individual behaviour;
4. differences in prioritization of long-term and short-term nursing objectives.

The most effective supervision of nursing practice is the one which shows respect for the ideas and opinions of others. However, it is also the role of the supervisor to guide the supervisee to a position of recognizing when extreme opinions are in conflict with the needs of the patient and the delivery of appropriate nursing care. Goal-setting may assist in producing a discussion and resolution of any differences, and may help both parties in seeing that they have generally more to agree about than to disagree. Supervisees may have to accept that a very modest treatment goal is not necessarily a negation of deeply-held principles, but simply a more realistic means of caring for the patient in the 'here and now'.

Important in this process of negotiation between supervisor and supervisee is effective communication. Matters which may seem like *affaires d'état* may frequently be due to the absence of a mutual language and a lack of listening to the latent content of what is being said. For the most part, sensitive handling can resolve these issues to the benefit of all concerned. There are, however, some occasions when it becomes necessary to acknowledge that fundamental differences in orientation do exist, and that the nurse concerned should seek supervision from someone more in tune with the way she interprets nursing practice. Nursing is a 'broad church', and there should be room for everyone, especially as there are different roads to the same end product.

Relationship

The supervisor's role is to assist the supervisee to apply theoretical knowledge, appropriate attitudes and the art of therapeutic communication to the treatment of patients. This is done primarily through the medium of the supervisory relationship as Platt-Kock (1986) writes:

'In supervision, the nurse gains theoretical knowledge but also learns to make new and fuller use of the self.'

This emphasis on self-awareness issues in supervision can sometimes serve to blur the boundaries, and supervisors may find themselves conducting a personal therapy rather than a supervision session.

Although supervision and psychotherapy are both helping processes, they differ significantly in their primary purpose and focus. Psychotherapy is about helping people to deal with inner conflicts and neurotic symptomatology. Supervision is about helping the nurse to increase her working skills more effectively with patients. Whilst this certainly involves more self-awareness, and the supervisor is involved in facilitating personal growth, the distinction between the therapeutic and supervisory relationship should be maintained. Platt-Koch (1986) refers to this similarity with psychotherapy and to the 'parallel process' which should be fostered but not exploited:

'Again there is a parallel to psychotherapy, in which the patient is helped to develop awareness of how thoughts and feelings affect behaviour. The patient can then make choices about how to live.'

The alliance between supervisor and supervisee is analogous to the therapeutic alliance, defined as the bond of trust between nurse and patient which is necessary for the practice of high quality nursing. By exploiting the emphasis on self-awareness issues in supervision, the supervisee may attempt to get 'therapy' from the supervisor, thereby diverting the sessions into a situation where personal needs are the centre of attention. Similarly, supervisors may wish to demonstrate their own understanding of the human psyche and may be guilty of over-analysing the responses of the supervisee, which often leads to resentment and anger. All these relationship 'traps' do nothing to serve the real purpose of supervision which is the promoting of learning about nursing, including some personal growth content.

Change is a difficult process for all of us, and at times the relationship in supervision can become 'stuck' in resistance to change which can take many forms, all usually related to difficulties experienced in the clinical situation with patients. Feeling comfortable with the idea of sharing one's work and feelings about it with a supervisor can also give rise to understandable sentiments of anxiety. Peplau (1957) contends that a certain optimum level of anxiety in the supervisory relationship is healthy and vitally necessary for any change or learning to take place. However, when these anxiety levels become too high, they must be addressed as they tend to interfere with learning and with the conduct of the supervision session. A common fantasy of supervisees is what might be termed the 'glass head syndrome' in which they come to believe early in a supervisory relationship that the more experienced, more qualified supervisor has the ability to know what is in their heads without them saying anything. That anxiety-provoking situation, if suspected, should be talked through. For Haller (1976), quality supervision depends on this ability of both parties to discuss the relationship itself when a problem prevents understanding and growth. And Platt-Koch (1986) sums up the relationship of supervision thus:

'Despite occasional problems, supervision should feel like a safe place for the nurse. Concomitantly, the supervisor should feel pleasure in nurturing a younger or less experienced clinician.'

Trust

Although this comes last in our description of the supervisory relationship, without trust there is no relationship. The supervisee, feeling exposed and without defences, must have absolute trust in the supervisor to keep them 'safe'. Reliability and consistency in word and action are important in providing an atmosphere in which the supervisee feels that the supervisor may be depended upon, whether this applies to commitments made for sessions or any other form of assistance. Essentially, one is aiming to provide what Rogerians describe as *unconditional positive regard* in the work situation. This means providing an atmosphere in which deficits in knowledge, attitudes or skills may be explored without being interpreted as a (negative) comment on the supervisee personally.

Closely linked to the development of such a climate is the sense of caring conveyed to supervisees by the time commitment and the energy invested on their behalf. Genuineness cannot be faked; the rule is: if you don't really care about the development of other nurses and nursing, don't become a supervisor, as it will only prove a persecutory relationship for those in your charge. Discussing trust in therapy, Dryden (1987) claims that one of our biggest problems lies in trusting ourselves:

> 'The person-centred approach is based on the belief that the human organism is trustworthy and that we have within us the necessary wisdom and resources for our development to full human-ness. And yet, how difficult it seems to be for those of us who are therapists to trust the truth of this assertion when we ourselves are the organism in question and when that organism is prompting in us a loving and spontaneous response to another person. Clearly, it is right and proper that we should be cautious for we know our capacity for self deception can be great.'

In affirming the supervisee's strengths, and recognizing the emotional demands of the nursing situation, the supervisor can make inroads into helping supervisees trust themselves and therefore others. As Middleman and Rhodes point out:

> 'In essence, by word and by deed, the supervisor contributes to the nurse's self-acceptance and confirmation.'

The establishment of trust also requires a high level of professionalism in the operation of supervisory boundaries. Supervision can place both parties in a strong transference situation. The intimate discussion of clinical and personal issues can, and should, have the effect, of producing closeness between supervisor and supervisee. Some inexperienced nurses may misinterpret the interest and concern of the supervisor or may openly express feelings of love and sexual attraction. These can be very difficult tests of trust and understanding for the sensitive supervisor who, whilst insisting on the retention of strictly professional boundaries, has no desire to hurt or humiliate the supervisee. The important learning experience for the latter is that sexual issues so often hidden in nursing can be discussed and the outcome remain positive. Trusting a supervisor with very intimate feelings without being overwhelmed by negative emotions can be an important learning experience. In the world of nursing, where we so often seem to pretend that gender and sexuality do not exist, it can come as a pleasant surprise to find out that a supervisor has human feelings.

In this chapter, we have attempted to provide a framework on which to base the supervisory relationship. By reference to a guide, such as the *growth and support* model, supervisors can ensure that all the essential elements of the relationship are given adequate emphasis. However, in presenting the model, we do not wish to imply that there is only one way of providing structure to the supervisory process. Supervision is, as we have stated, a personal as well as professional experience, and it is precisely this human element which allows for the great breadth and variety of approach.

REFERENCES

Balint, M. (1957) *The Doctor, His Patient, and The Illness*, Int. University Press, New York.

Barber, P. and Norman, I. (1987) Mental Health Nursing. Skills in supervision, *Nursing Times*, 14 Jan., **83**(2), 56–7.

Bion, W. R. (1975) *Brazilian lectures*, 1. Imago Editora, Rio de Janeiro.

Brammer, L. M. and Wassmer A. C. (1977) Supervision in counselling and psychotherapy, in Kurpius, D. J. (ed.) *et al.*, *Supervision of Applied Training: A Comparative Review*, Greenwood Press, London.

Burnard, P. (1988) Mentors: A supporting act, *Nursing Times*. 16 Nov., **84**(46).

Casement, P. (1985) *On Learning From the Patient*, Tavistock, London.

Darling, L. A. W. (1984) What do nurses want in a mentor? *Journal of Nursing Administration*. Oct., **14**(10), 42–4.

Dryden, W. (1987) *Key Cases in Psychotherapy*, Croom Helm, London.

Ekstein, R. and Wallenstein, R. S. (1958) *The Teaching and Learning of Psychotherapy*, Int. University Press, New York.

Haller, L. L. (1976) Clinical psychiatric supervision. Process and problems. A method of teaching psychiatric concepts in nursing education, *Perspective in Psychiatric Care*, **14**, 115–29.

Halgin, R. P. (1986) Pragmatic blending of clinical model in the supervision relationship, *The Clinical Supervisor*, **3**, (Winter 85–86), 23–46.

Hobson, R. (1985) *Forms of Feeling: The Heart of Psychotherapy*, Tavistock, London.

Ivey, A. (1977) Foreword, in Kurpius, D. J. *et al.*, *Supervision of Applied Training. A Comparative Review*, Greenwood Press, London.

Kadushin, A. (1976) *Supervision in Social Work*, Columbia Press, New York.

Langs, R. (1979) *The Supervisory Experience*, Aronson, New York.

Malan, D. H. (1975) *A Study of Brief Psychotherapy*, Plenum Rosetta, New York.

McCarthy, P. (1985) Burnout in psychiatric nursing, *Journal of Advanced Nursing*, **10**, 305–10.

McFarlane, J. (1982) Nursing values and nursing action, *Nursing Times*. 29 Sept., **78**(39), 109–12.

Menzies, I. E. P. (1960) *Nurses Under Stress: A Social System Functioning as a Defence Against Anxiety*, Tavistock pamphlet no. 3, Tavistock, London.

Middleman, R. and Rhodes, G. (1985) *Competent Supervision: Making Imaginative Judgements*, Prentice-Hall, New Jersey.

Pembrey, S. (1980) *The Ward Sister, Key to Nursing*, RCN, London.

Peplau, H. E. (1957) What is experiential teaching? *American Journal of Nursing*, 884–6.

Pettes, D. E. (1979) *Staff and Student Supervision: A Staff Centered Approach*, Allen & Unwin, London.

Platt-Kock, L. M. (1986) Clinical supervision for psychiatric nurses, *Journal of Psycho-social Nursing*, January, **26**(1), 7–15.

Puetz, B. E. (1985) Learn the ropes from a mentor. *Nursing Success Today*, **2**(6), 11–13.

Seebohm, F. (1968) *Report of Committee on Local Authority and Personal and Social Services*, HMSO, London.

Watts, G. (1987) *Clinical Supervision in Community Psychiatric Nursing*, unpublished report, Leeds University.

Westheimer, I. (1977) *The Practice of Supervision in Social Work. A Guide for Supervisors*, Ward Lock Educational, London.

Wolberg, L. R. (1988) *The Teaching of Psychotherapy*, 4th edition, Part 2, Grune & Stratton, New York.

Wright, S. G. (1986) *Building and Using a Model of Nursing*, Edward Arnold, London.

The therapeutic use of self | 3

David Woods

INTRODUCTION

Peter was a nurse working in a hospice. He had worked there for four years and was proud that no other member of staff had worked in the unit for as long and with as little time off for sickness as he had. He had seen other members of staff come and stay for a year or two and then leave to work in other branches of nursing. He had supported and cared for a great many patients and had helped them to die with dignity.

In one of the hospice unit's weekly staff support groups he became very upset and disturbed one day and described a recurring dream that he had almost every night. The dream made him feel frightened and anxious for his future. He could not make sense of it and brought it to the group because he was at the end of his tether. This was unusual for Peter, because although he didn't openly scorn the group he didn't think he needed it. In his recurrent dream he was walking down a corridor with doors on either side. He felt compelled to go into each room and in each room lying in bed dying was a member of his own family, reaching out to him for help. He described feeling that he wanted to kill them and as he walked towards them to suffocate them he woke up. This left him feeling distressed and uncomfortable and not knowing what the dream meant to him.

When he discussed it in the group, one or two members recognized that the dream was more about his work in the hospice than it was a dream about his family. They were able to give him feedback about the way he was apparently able to tolerate the stress and distress of working in the unit. They were able to reflect back to him that he never seemed to be upset on duty when people died. Peter was able to share with them for the first time his anxieties about working in the unit and his increasing personal distress about wanting to distance himself from people who came on to the unit, feeling that if he nursed them they surely would die.

Over the following months Peter was able to talk more openly about the distress of the deaths of so many people on the unit and eventually decided to leave the unit to work in another branch of nursing. He left with a sense of achievement and was looking forward to the future rather than leaving feeling that he could not cope, which is what had prevented him from leaving before.

Jane had been feeling miserable and depressed for a number of months. She had been feeling increasingly unwell and despondent about her life. She was able to identify the beginnings of her feelings of unhappiness and sadness as starting about the time that her daughter, now aged nine months old, was born. She talked over her symptoms and feelings with her general practitioner and they both agreed that her difficult feelings were related to the birth of her child and that she would probably get over it in time. The general practitioner rightly said to her that if she didn't feel much better she must come back and talk things through with him. Jane didn't feel any better. She felt more depressed and upset about her husband, feeling that he didn't understand her and that his work was more important in his life than either she or their daughter was.

Jane returned to her general practitioner and they talked through what had been happening to her. He was keen that they shouldn't seek a pharmacological solution to her problems and that she needed the opportunity to resolve both her relationship with her husband and her feelings about the birth of her child. They agreed that it might be helpful for Jane to see somebody regularly to work through her feelings. The general practitioner arranged that Jane came to see a nurse who was attached to the health centre on a weekly basis.

Jane came every week and spent an hour discussing her feelings and her difficulties. The nurse for her part encouraged Jane to express the feelings that she had and helped her to get in touch with her difficulties. As the sessions continued, Jane felt, for the first time in her life, that someone understood the difficulties that she had and understood her predicament. She eventually decided that her marriage was no longer sustainable. She felt that there were so many differences between her and her husband and that she could no longer continue. She was worried about having made this decision, but was encouraged and supported in her decision by the nurse. The nurse understood and was able to reflect back to Jane that it was difficult, but would probably help her more in the long run. After several months of therapy, Jane did get divorced and finished her therapy, no longer feeling the need to discuss her feelings. The nurse for her part felt that a good job had been done. Jane had taken more responsibility for her life and, with a lot of help, had made an appropriate decision about ending her marriage.

Three months later Jane returned to her general practitioner chronically depressed and unable to function. She felt in danger of physically abusing her child. She felt she had made an enormous mistake in getting divorced and wasn't sure which way to turn next. The general practitioner discussed it in passing with the nurse who had seen Jane for so many months. The nurse remarked, 'I really don't know why it didn't work for her. When I had my baby and got depressed I was in just the same position as her and my divorce was the making of me. I wonder why it wasn't for her?'

What is important about these two simple illustrations is that the feelings, anxieties, thoughts and expressions of emotion of the two nurses, both acknowledged and unacknowledged, had a bearing and an influence on the quality of the relationship and affected the outcome of the care. Jane presented in extreme distress and sought help for that distress. The outcome and apparent resolution of that distress was not what she really wanted. It is possible to hypothesize that the formulation and conceptualization of Jane's difficulties and the understanding of the way to resolve them was largely shaped by the nurse's own personal experience rather than from a clear understanding of Jane's position. It is clear that the solution of separation and divorce may have been appropriate for the nurse. It is not so clear that it was appropriate for Jane. It left her feeling angry at herself for taking the advice, but also let down and depressed about the position she was in, which she felt was worse than the position she had started with.

In the first illustration, Peter contained his feelings and did not acknowledge they had any importance in the work he was doing. The denial of his own upset and distress at the painful work he was doing overflowed into his life outside of work and caused him great anxiety. The danger for Peter and his patients, had he not articulated his difficulties, would have been that he increasingly distanced himself from his patients because he was frightened that he would act out his murderous fantasies.

All nursing activity takes place in the context of a human relationship. That relationship may be a brief, concise and contained relationship which may occur with someone attending an accident and emergency department, or it may be a more complex, ongoing relationship between a nurse and a patient over a long period of time in a ward or in the community.

It is important for nurses to recognize and value the uniqueness of this human relationship between people. Whatever branch of nursing is chosen, whether it be the nursing of people who are physically sick or people who suffer from poor mental health, it is important to acknowledge the feelings, fantasies and experiences that the nurse brings to the relationship.

Everyone has a life history and the way in which we behave and react and, more importantly, interact in our daily lives is moulded and informed by the personal psychological experiences we have had in our lives. When the nurse interacts and communicates with a patient, we cannot and should not deny the internal world or the life experiences of the nurse. Nursing is not an impersonal relationship where the patient is reduced to the position of being a powerless child in relation to the doctor representing the dominant father, and the nurse acting as mother compliantly servicing the family and carrying out father's wishes. Patients are active, thoughtful, reflective, feeling beings with an equal share in the relationship, however vulnerable and fragile their illness leaves them feeling.

If nurses are to maintain and improve the quality of their relationships with their patients they must make greater effort to enhance the use of their feelings and emotions. This therapeutic use of the self is central to a living dynamic relationship.

Creating and maintaining a relationship which is ultimately going to be helpful to the patient in restoring him or her to as healthy a position as possible is not something which comes by chance. The reality is that there are more likely to be problems with maintaining that relationship. These problems can perhaps be discussed in three areas:

- organizational structure;
- occupational stress;
- professionalism.

ORGANIZATIONAL STRUCTURE

The way in which nurses function, and the way in which their relationships with their patients develop, must be taken in the context of the organizational structure in which they exist. Undoubtedly the managerial and economic climate in which health care takes place has changed radically over the last five to ten years. There is a great emphasis on managerialism and an increasingly centralized control of health care (Best, 1987), accompanied by an increased emphasis on 'productivity and throughput'. The length of stay in hospital is shorter, community services are increasingly burdened with large numbers of patients who have been discharged after even shorter stays. Resources are in reality scarcer (Klien, 1985). Demand for health-care expenditure has exceeded resource availability (DHSS, 1983; Gamble and Walkland, 1984; Klein, 1985). Nursing in the 1980s saw a major reorganization, with in 1982 a change in its management system, with the introduction of general management in 1983–4, and the biggest restructuring and reorganization of its nursing services ever with clinical grading from 1988 onwards. The 1990s brought the reforms of the NHS and community care provision.

At the same time there has been great emphasis placed on quality assurance, personalizing the service and consumer choice. Not, however, without a great deal of criticism. The main critics claim that the increased emphasis on consumer choice and personal services are little more than a 'supermarket window-dressing'.

This climate of increased managerialism and cash limiting of services imposes tremendous stresses on nurses attempting to have an open helpful relationship with their patients. The danger is that many aspects of nursing care are simply impossible to carry out. Constraints on time and external pressures impose impossible demands. In busy acute wards it is quite common for nurses to return from their two days off and not know any of the patients on their ward. The question must seriously be asked, what is this doing to the ability of the nurse to care appropriately and adequately for the patient? It must feel quite impossible at times to pay attention to the psychological meaning of relationships when there are so many external pressures.

Often, general managers and nurse managers are neither equipped nor sufficiently experienced to understand the importance of creating a culture and structure for care which supports and enhances the ability of nurses. In her classic work, Isobel Menzies (1959) was highly critical of the way in which nursing services were organized, and hypothesized that they were structured to avoid the personal interaction that took place between nurses and patients and that this was designed to avoid the internal anxiety engendered by intimacy of the relationship.

Interestingly, not to say sadly, Menzies Lyth (1988) has more recently expressed that although some things have changed she does not really perceive any major differences in the present day organization of nursing, and would appear to be critical of the pursuit of professionalization. She argues that nurses require opportunity to understand their personal feelings, perceptions and anxieties about their work; in a sense more opportunity for tea and talk rather than yet another reorganization and higher professional qualifications.

There are some examples of improvements in the way in which nursing is organized and the way in which nurses conceptualize their work. Attempts have been made to schematize the needs of patients into the nursing process and, at the same time, by attempting to use models nurses have attempted more clearly to understand and identify patients' needs. Unfortunately, these models and processes often focus on the individual patient and do not attempt to understand interactions in the context of a relationship. There is an almost universal denial that the nurse's actions, feelings and perceptions of the patient are of any importance. This is equally true in psychiatric nursing with its residual emphasis on organic medical models of mental disease.

The world of modern nursing with its processes, models, high technology, efficiency and output is a very difficult place for the nurse who wishes to emphasize the healing process and values the skills of nurturing, caring and compassion.

OCCUPATIONAL STRESS

Nursing is often a painful business and the pain experienced by nurses in carrying out their day-to-day work often goes unacknowledged, at great personal cost. Several authors (Maslach, 1976, Maslach and Jackson, 1981, Gowler and Parry, 1983) have identified stress as one of the major reasons why nurses fail to function. Parry and Gowler have identified the *cruciform effect* as being directly related to stress in the caring professions. They describe a situation where conflicting values exert pressures upon professionals. Professionals with a basic mandate to provide a personal service (the basic mandate in the case of nursing is personal care) may find this mandate directly and indirectly challenged by organizational priorities. The organizational priorities require the professional to respond to other considerations. Briefly stated, the cruciform effect occurs where the individual worker is unable to resolve internally the tension between their basic mandate and the priority constructed by the organization. This inability to tolerate the tension results in four types of coping behaviours:

- *easing* – nurses who ease reduce their contact time with patients, spending considerably more time looking after their colleagues, organizing administrative duties, editing books or journals, or acting as nurse consultants;
- *freezing* – this is basically a denial of the difficulty of the relationship. Freezers close their eyes to the real world and suffering of their patients. They are very careful to select patients who will get better and accept the professionals limited view of care. They tend to be over-cautious and slavishly follow procedures. It is doubtful, though, whether they help many people;
- *seizing* – seizers avoid patients by embracing new technologies and techniques which enable them to reformulate the complexity of the human being into a series of technical problems. The ultimate expression of seizing may be retreating into research well away from patient contact;
- *melting* – this is a result of internal stress. This complex and ambivalent form of coping involves a dissolving of relationships with more conventional colleagues. Melters are radical nurses who are only too aware of the discomfort of the cruciform effect. They are vociferous in their criticism of easers, freezers and seizers. This method of coping is in direct contrast to freezing and presents itself as a form of interprofessional tension. Melters attempt to resolve the stresses by turning away from conventional one-to-one relationships and try to interact directly with the community. They disown professional skill and status. However, they very rarely disown professional salary, but nearly

always remain on the payroll of a conservative organization. The dilemma of the melter is rarely resolved.

These descriptions are not intended to be disparaging but more an indication of the complex way in which individuals cope with the stress placed upon them by their painful work.

Menzies, as indicated above, has identified that the very organization of services enables nurses to defend against the anxiety that is generated by their work. This defence is both organizational and personal: organizational in that the structure legislates against the intimacy of nursing relationships developing fully; and personally, because as Menzies points out, if the individual rejects the organizational defence system and continues to use his or her own, there is a risk of rejection from colleagues. In adopting the organizational defence system there will be an increase in anxiety which might result in nurses finding themselves unable to continue any further. This interface between individuals' feelings and the way in which nursing is organized creates constant pressure for the individual. Menzies Lyth (1988) noted almost 30 years after her original work that wastage rates for nurses in training are not significantly different now from 1959.

PROFESSIONALISM

The pursuit of professional status for nurses may well legislate against the creation and maintenance of helpful relationships with patients. Some writers (Navarro, 1976; Illich, 1977; Doyle, 1979; Wilding, 1982) have stated that the pursuit of professional status may compromise the defined aim of the profession and do more for members of the profession than it does for the clients it seeks to serve.

The professionalization of nursing and its consequences require further discussion if some understanding of the implications are to be recognized for the quality of nursing relationships.

A profession can be defined as an occupational group which has a legally supported monopoly by a registration system. In the case of nurses this is the United Kingdom Central Council and the 1979 Nurses, Midwives and Health Visitors Act. An occupational group which is able to control its own work, educational standards, entry into the profession, has professional autonomy over practice, and, perhaps most importantly, is only open to scrutiny by its peers, is a very powerful group. How this power is used is open to examination.

Johnson (1972) says that one of the main characteristics of a profession is the social distance and the unequal relationship between the professional and the clients, or, simply stated, he said that the more an occupational group seeks professional status, the more it becomes socially distanced from its clients and recreates the inequality of society in the professional–client relationship. Is the creation of an asymmetrical relationship what is really needed in nurse–patient relationships?

If nursing, as it would appear to do, is intent on pursuing the aim of professionalization, then there are inherent dangers. Much of nursing activity and nursing relationships should focus on a sense of 'being with' the patient, that is holding and containing the patient's anxiety for them and being with them when they are at their most vulnerable. In professionalized relationships there is often an over emphasis on 'doing to'. In these relationships, there is focus on technical expertise and practical procedures, which do not always take account of the patient's primitive anxiety.

The pursuit of professionalization creates great pressure on nurses and may well militate against them having a helpful, caring, nurturing relationship with patients.

CREATING THE ENVIRONMENT TO USE SELF

For nurses to use their life experiences appropriately they need to give appropriate regard to the environment in which nursing activity takes place. Creating an appropriate environment is broader than simply ensuring an appropriate physical environment, it is also about creating the appropriate psychological environment. The way in which the psychological environment or space is created is important. The use of the word 'space' in this context is deliberate. It acknowledges that personal psychological space to explore the internal feelings and anxieties that are created by being vulnerable and ill is as important as the technical and practical procedures.

The psychological space should lead the nurse to understand her position in the relationship. It should lead to the questions: Why am I interacting in this way? Why did I say this in preference to that? What are my feelings in the relationship and what feelings belong to the patient? In order for the feelings and experiences of the nurses to be understandable they need to placed within a framework which informs practice. There are numerous theoretical psychological models to inform practice, and arguments will continue about which is the most appropriate. What is important is the ability to find a consistent model for oneself which is comfortable and allows understanding to develop.

Winnicott (1971; Davis and Wallbridge, 1981) had a clear framework for his work as a paediatrician. He was able to describe a psychological framework for his activity during a consultation with a mother and a child. Rather than just focus on the activity of the mother or of the child, he was able to describe a framework that recognized the relationship between himself as a paediatrician and the mother and child. In his work he created a psychological space with clearly defined boundaries that allowed the mother and child to experience their relationship and to work through the difficult and painful feelings that relationship engendered. This framework prevented Winnicott from intervening prematurely when it might have been inappropriate. It may have been that to intervene would have prevented the resolution of the feelings that both mother and child had in the relationship. Winnicott described the mother as physically *holding* the child and he (the doctor) psychologically *holding* the situation. Holding is a way of containing the anxiety created in relationships and provides a way of understanding the process.

Similarly within nursing it is often the ward sister who psychologically holds the situation on the ward and often the staff nurse and health-care assistant who physically holds (nurtures/nurses) the patient. Holding does not take place by accident – it is a combination of organizational structure, an internalization of theory and a recognition of the position of the self in the relationship. The actions of the nurse are informed by the process of holding, rather than being acted out in response to the content of the patient's internal world and projections.

The actions of the nurse in the relationship should take into account the feelings of the patient as well as the feelings that are being felt but not acknowledged by the nurse. For example, Susan, a speech therapist was a patient in the maternity unit following the birth of her first child. Sadly, the child was born with a cleft palate and a hare lip. Susan was clearly upset, but more distressed to find that no one came to talk to her about it and she was moved to a side room. She eventually read her case notes, which were left casually at the bottom of her bed. Written in large red letters at the top of the page was 'mother is anxious + + +'. Susan asked the staff nurse who looked after her why she had said that she was anxious about the cleft palate and hair lip when she had not discussed it with her. The staff nurse felt unable to explain her 'diagnosis' of anxiety but felt that because Susan was a speech therapist it must be impossible for her to bear the upset of her child's 'deformity'. She went on to say that she knew very little about the child's problems and prognosis. What is apparent is that the feelings that the staff nurse had about the child made her prejudge the situation. What would have been more appropriate would have been for her to acknowledge her own feelings about the baby and sit down with Susan to discuss hers. The staff nurse's own anxious feelings made Susan feel isolated and unsupported at a time of great stress. In this case, the feelings of the nurse were clearly projected onto the patient. It was not possible for the nurse to recognize which feelings belonged to her and which feelings belonged to the patient.

Sometimes the feelings that nurses have during interactions are positively helpful in helping the patient to understand their position and difficulties. Stephen was being seen by a community psychiatric nurse (CPN) on a weekly basis. He was 17 and living at home with his parents. He was referred because he was 'depressed and isolated'. He came along week after week, nothing apparently changing. The CPN found Stephen an increasingly irritating patient who made him feel angry because he wouldn't change. Stephen seemed unable to generate any enthusiasm for anything. The CPN did not express his angry feelings in the sessions with the patient, but discussed them in supervision. The supervisor and the nurse reflected on the meaning of the nurse's feelings and, more importantly, on what they might mean in the context of the CPN's relationship with Stephen. At the next session the nurse said to Stephen that he felt angry at him at times in the sessions. Stephen, who usually had his head down, looked up, smiled and said 'My dad always says that'. Over the subsequent sessions, Stephen was able to talk more about his relationship with his father. He said that as far as his father was concerned he was a failure and Stephen felt that nothing he could do or say would change that. Stephen described his intense feelings of anger at his father which previously had not been recognized or expressed. Stephen was slowly able to liberate himself from his painful feelings by exploring them in a safe, contained, structured environment. The recognition of the angry feelings in the nurse and the structured exploration of them allowed Stephen to express how he really felt. The recreation of his relationship with his father in the relationship with the CPN allowed Stephen to understand his anger about his father's disappointment, rather than simply acting it out as depression. As he became able to express his angry feeling directly to his father, he no longer needed to feel depressed and isolated.

The appropriate recognition of the nurse's own feelings, the framework to understand those feelings and the ability to contain those feelings allowed a clear understanding of the difficulties that the patient was experiencing.

TOWARDS SELF-AWARENESS

Becoming self-aware and being able to make good use of the self-awareness is not something which automatically occurs. Indeed, several writers have reflected on the difficulty of teaching good communication skills in nursing practice (Faulkner *et al.*, 1983; Hein, 1980; Mcleod Clarke, 1981). Nor is it appropriate to assume that self-awareness development is only important in basic training; there has to be consistent ongoing development of self-awareness throughout professional practice.

As nurses develop in their career, they move from being anxious about their relationships and ability to a position of greater confidence. In this position of confidence,they are more able to tolerate the uncertainty and ambiguity of their role. The more experience and training nurses have, the less they feel they know. In nursing practice this is something that should be cultivated, rather than something to be afraid of.

It is not really realistic to expect that each individual nurse should bear the whole responsibility for their individual practice alone. The nurse is in a context and in a relationship with patients, colleagues and the organization he or she works for. It is important to think about the development of self-awareness in broader terms than focusing on the individual. It is perhaps helpful to consider three prerequisites which might need to be met before self-awareness can develop fully:

- *Organizational culture* – It will not be possible to develop and use one's own feelings and experiences if the organizational culture that one is operating in is not receptive. If the idea that nurses' feelings should not be expressed is the dominant cultural norm then any expression of emotion is going to be frowned upon. The development of a culture which values the personal feelings, experiences and emotions of its nurses is not just the responsibility of one person. The whole organization must share the same cultural values and norms.
- *A structured way of thinking about the relationship and the interaction* – There are many frameworks and models for conceptualizing the meaning of the interaction and informing an appropriate response. Often these models, whether they be psychoanalytic, behavioural or cognitive, are seen as competing and different. Rather than using a multitude of models it is often more sensible to use one that 'psychologically fits' the nurse. If a model or framework 'fits' it makes sense and is comfortable for the nurse. Smith (1979; 1986) has outlined a useful framework to help student psychiatric nurses understand process and content of their relationships. This helpful framework has wider application in all branches of nursing.
- *Constant and consistent supervision* – This is perhaps the most important element in enabling the use of self in the nursing relationship. The function of supervision is to enable and facilitate the process of the nursing relationship. It should not be seen as a hierarchical, controlling relationship.

SUMMARY

This chapter has focused on the therapeutic use of self in the nursing relationship. The importance of acknowledging the context in which the relationship takes place has been discussed as well as the limitations in terms of organizational structure, occupational stress and the pursuit of professionalization of nursing. The broad way in which the environmental conditions have to be correct and created to use self are discussed. Finally, there is a brief description of the prerequisites for making appropriate use of self in the nurse–patient relationship.

REFERENCES

Best, G. (1987) *The Future of NHS General Management: Where Next?* King's Fund Centre, London.

Davis, M. and Wallbridge, D. (1981) *Boundary and Space: An Introduction to the Work of D. W. Winnicott*, Karnac, London.

DHSS (1983) *Health Care and its Costs*, HMSO, London.

Doyle, L. (1979) *The Political Economy of Health*, Pluto Press, London.

Faulkner, A., Bridge, W., Macleod Clarke, J. and Williams, A. (1983) *Teaching Communication Skills in Nursing*, Paper given at RCN Research Conference, Brighton.

Gamble, A. M. and Walkland, S. A. (1984) *The British Party System and Economic Policy 1945–1983*, Clarendon Press, London.

Gowler, D. and Parry, G. (1983) Career stresses on psychological therapists, in Pilgrim, D. (ed.) *Psychology and Psychotherapy. Current Trends and Issues*, Routledge & Kegan Paul, London.

Hein, E. C. (1980) *Communication in Nursing Practice*, Little Brown, Boston.

Illich, I. (1977) *Limits to Medicine. Medical Nemesis: The Expropriation of Health*, Penguin, London.

Johnson, T. J. (1972) *Professions and Power*, Macmillan, London.

Klein, R. (1985) 'Health Policy 1979–1983: The retreat from ideology?, in Jackson, P. M. (ed.) *Implementing Government Policy Initiatives*, RIPA, London.

Macleod Clarke, J. (1981) Communication in nursing, *Nursing Times*, **77**(1), 12–18.

Maslach, C. (1976) Burned out, *Human Behaviour*, **5**, 16–22.

Maslach, C. and Jackson, S. E. (1981) Measurement of experienced burnout, *Journal of Occupational Behaviour*, **2**, 99–113.

Menzies, I. E. P. (1959) The functioning of social systems as a defence against anxiety: A report on a study of the nursing service of a general hospital, *Human Relations*, **13**, 95–121.

Menzies Lyth, I. E. P. (1988) *Containing Anxiety in Institutions: Selected Essays*, Free Association Books, London.

Navarro, V. (1976) *Medicine under Capitalism*, Prodist, New York.

Smith, L. (1979) Communication skills, *Nursing Times*, **75**(22), 926–9.

Smith, L. (1986) Talking it out, *Nursing Times*, **82**(13), 38–43.

Wilding, P. (1982) *Professional Power and Social Welfare*, Routledge & Kegan Paul, London.

Winnicott, D. W. (1971) *Therapeutic Consultations in Child Psychiatry*, Hogarth Press, London.

Clinical supervision, stress management and social support

4

Jerome Carson, Tony Butterworth and Katie Booth

INTRODUCTION

In the first edition, we reviewed the literature on stress in nursing and discussed how nursing staff might be better supported in their work. In this chapter we summarize findings from two empirical studies that have addressed these issues directly. The first study set out to evaluate the effects of a social support based intervention with mental health nurses using a randomized controlled design. The second study, the Clinical Supervision Evaluation Project, is the most ambitious study yet conducted into the effects of clinical supervision on nursing staff. In this chapter we present some data that attempt to answer the question of whether clinical supervision has a beneficial effect on the mental well-being of nurses and health visitors. The evidence for social support and clinical supervision is far from convincing. Finally we make some general comments on stress management for nursing staff.

STUDY 1: THE BETHLEM MAUDSLEY NURSING STRESS INTERVENTION STUDY

Introduction

Research evidence has been accumulating steadily on stress in nursing (Grey-Toft and Anderson, 1981; Hipwell *et al.*, 1989; Wheeler, 1997), while fewer studies have been conducted into stress in mental health nurses (Dawkins *et al.*, 1985; Fagin *et al.*, 1996). The studies that have been conducted suggest that mental health nursing is also stressful. Indeed, there is evidence from America that mental health nurses sustain more injuries from violent incidents at work than workers in occupations that are known as high risk, such as construction and forestry (Love and Hunter, 1996). The annual injury rate per 100 employees is 8.3 for mining, 13.1 for manufacturing, 14.2 for heavy construction, 18.4 for forestry and 22.4 for nursing. Violence is only one of the problems that face mental health nurses. The key question is: Can anything be done to reduce stress levels in mental health nurses? This study aimed to address this issue.

The wider literature on coping with stress highlights the importance of social support as a coping technique (Pierce *et al.*, 1997). A number of studies report that there is an inverse relationship between social support and occupational stress. Staff who lack social support experience greater distress that those with adequate support networks (Cronin-Stubbs and Brophy, 1985). However, some nurse researchers claim that social support has a negligible effect on staff stress (Norbeck, 1985). To date, no researcher has conducted a randomized, controlled trial of the efficacy of social support as a moderator of stress in mental health nurses.

The intervention utilized in this study was developed over a number of years by the first author (see an early description of a pilot study by Ritter *et al.*, 1995). The rationale behind the intervention is that social support is an effective moderator of stress. The initial pilot study used a quasi-experimental design to show that the programme was more effective than a no-treatment control. The programme has also been shown to be effective with a group of long-term unemployed, though it was not as effective as cognitive therapy (Proudfoot *et al.*, 1997). The programme aimed to capitalize on findings such as the positive therapeutic benefits of belonging to groups (Yalom, 1985) and the development of psychoeducational approaches (Wycherley, 1987). Rather than have a no-treatment control condition, it was decided to conduct a randomized, controlled trial of the social support condition versus a feedback condition.

Method

The sample was drawn from ward-based mental health nurses at the Bethlem and Maudsley Hospitals. Out of the 64 nurses who volunteered, 53 completed the batch of questionnaires, enabling them to be randomized – a response rate of 82 per cent. Of these, 36 per cent were male, 51 per cent were staff nurses and a further 30 per cent were charge nurse grade or above. Participants ranged in age from 22 to 51 years and had worked in nursing for an average of 7.68 years and had been in their present job for an average of 1.84 years. After random allocation, the Social Support Group had 27 participants and the Feedback Group 26. An advertisement describing the project was placed in the hospital bulletin and fliers were sent to all wards. Presentations were made to ward managers, and all wards were visited individually by the research team. Volunteers were seen individually and asked to sign consent forms and then to complete the study questionnaires. Random allocation was carried out by sealed envelope, utilizing random permuted blocks.

All participants completed the following questionnaires:

- *Demographic Questionnaire*: this had 29 items, covering age, grade, sex, etc.
- *The General Health Questionnaire*: We used the 28-item form (Goldberg and Williams, 1988). This is the most widely used psychiatric screening tool worldwide (Bowling, 1995). Two principal measures are obtained, these are Total GHQ score and 'Caseness' score, scores of five or more on this version.
- *The Maslach Burnout Inventory*: Developed by Maslach and Jackson (1986), this assesses occupational burnout syndrome. Scores are obtained on the three independent components of burnout, namely Emotional Exhaustion, Depersonalization and Personal Accomplishment. In addition to scores for each subscale, categorical scores are given for each subscale, classifying individuals as having high, moderate or low burnout on each dimension.
- *The DeVilliers, Carson, Leary Stress Scale (The DCL Stress Scale)*: This is a measure of stress developed specifically for ward-based mental health nurses. Five factor scores are obtained: Patient Demands, Organizational and Managerial Issues, Staffing, Future Concerns and Job Satisfaction. A Total DCL Stress Score is also obtained. (Copies of the DCl can be obtained by writing to the first author.)
- *The Rosenberg Self-Esteem Scale*: A 10 item scale that measures individuals' levels of self-esteem (Rosenberg, 1965).
- *The Pearlin Mastery Scale*: A seven-item scale that measures the extent to which individuals see themselves as being in control of the forces that affect their lives (Pearlin and Schooler, 1978).
- *The Cooper Coping Skills Scale*: This scale examines the frequency of use of a range of coping skills. It has six subscales covering social support, task organization, logic, home and work relationships, time management and involvement with work aims. Subscale scores and a total score are obtained. It is part of the wider Occupational Stress Indicator (Cooper *et al.*, 1988).
- *The Significant Others Scale (Short Version)*: This questionnaire measures social support by examining the relationships with spouse/partner, mother, father, sibling, child, best friend (Power *et al.*, 1988). It examines two types of support, emotional and practical, and it gives an actual and ideal rating.

- *The Minnesota Job Satisfaction Scale*: This has 20 items that assess Intrinsic, Extrinsic and Total Job Satisfaction (Weiss *et al.*, 1967).
- *The Eysenck Personality Questionnaire (EPQ-R Short Scale)*: The short form of the EPQ was used (Eysenck and Eysenck, 1991). This covers the three core dimensions of Personality, Extroversion, Neuroticism, Psychoticism. It also has a built in Lie Scale.

Participants who were randomized into the Social Support Intervention were required to attend five two-hour group sessions facilitated by a senior nurse and an assistant psychologist, held at weekly intervals. Sessions were held in the training centres of both hospitals. Sessions followed a set format. At the beginning of each meeting an overview was given, and then any outstanding issues from the previous session were discussed. The exercises for that particular session were completed by all of the participants including the facilitators. Confidentiality was stressed. At the end of each session an evaluation was conducted. Task assignments relating to specific topics were given each week, to be completed before the next session. A brief outline of the themes covered in each of the five sessions is given below:

- *Session 1*: Introductions. Warm-up exercise. An examination of work stressors. The rationale for the intervention and background evidence for the social support model.
- *Session 2*: Graph of personal life satisfaction. This was completed by each participant and each person then fed-back their own graph to the group. This highlights the link between life events and stress. The assignment focused on an individual who helped the person cope with a major transitional stressor.
- *Session 3*: Social role mapping. Participants reported on their major life roles, ranked these in order of importance, and then rated their satisfaction with each of these. Participants were asked to think about who supported them in their main social roles.
- *Session 4*: Each participant was asked to draw up their own social support network and to feed this back. The issue of social popularity was covered. The task assignment examined the rules of social relationships and required participants to establish the key rules for a close personal relationship and a close friendship.
- *Session 5*: Goal-setting comprised the main item for the last session. Participants were required to answer the questions: What social support do I need? Who is going to give me that support? How will I get that support? How am I going to make sure that happens? Goals were again fed-back to each other. Participants were then asked to make positive comments about each other on 'Post-it' notes. The facilitators then summarized the main points of the intervention and linked

the five sessions. The session ended with the completion of a second batch of questionnaires and a feedback form.

Those staff randomized into the Feedback Only Group were contacted approximately five weeks after completion of the first set of questionnaires. Each participant was visited in their place of work and their questionnaire results explained verbally, to enable any queries to be answered. They also received a copy of their results and a booklet on stress management tips compiled by the researchers. A fortnight after receiving their feedback, the participants were asked to complete a second batch of questionnaires.

All participants in both the Social Support and Feedback Groups were therefore assessed prior to randomization, after the treatment condition was concluded and then again after six months. As mentioned earlier, 27 staff were allocated to Social Support. Three of these did not attend any sessions. Hence 24 received this intervention. At the six-month follow-up, 17 of these were reassessed – 71 per cent. Some 26 staff were allocated to Feedback Only and 23 of these were assessed post-intervention. At the six month follow-up, 17 of these were reassessed – 74 per cent. The main reason for attrition was staff leaving the organization.

Results

The results of the study will be presented in the format of the stress model developed by Carson and Kuipers (1998). The model postulates three levels of the stress process:

1 *Stressors*: The only measure that directly tapped into stressors was the DCL Stress Sale.
2 *Moderators of the Stress Process*: These were the Eysenck Personality Questionnaire, the Rosenberg Self-Esteem Scale, the Pearlin Scale, the Cooper Coping Skills Scale, and the Significant Others scale.
3 *Stress Outcomes*: These were assessed by the General Health Questionnaire, the Maslach Burnout Inventory, the Minnesota Job Satisfaction Scale and items from the Demographic Scale such as sickness absence.

Stressors

There were no significant differences in stressors on the DCL Scale between both groups at pre- or post-intervention (see Table 4.1). However, by the time of the six month follow-up the Feedback Group had significantly lower stress scores on Patient Demands, Organizational and Managerial stress and on the DCL Total Stress Score. Within both groups there was a trend towards lower stress over time.

Table 4.1. DCL Stress Scores from the Bethlem Maudsley Nursing Stress Intervention Study

Subscale	Pre-intervention	Post-intervention	Follow-up
Patient demands:			
Social Support	15.52 (5.36)	16.00 (5.64)	15.65 (4.65)
Feedback	13.77 (6.17)	13.39 (4.65)	9.76 (3.25) p < 0.001
Organizational and Managerial:			
Social Support	15.22 (5.50)	15.36 (6.09)	14.47 (5.30)
Feedback	13.42 (7.11)	12.74 (6.67)	10.53 (4.92) p < 0.05
Staffing:			
Social Support	15.07 (5.43)	14.24 (5.58)	13.35 (4.43)
Feedback	12.73 (5.63)	11.39 (5.14)	11.17 (5.19)
Future concerns:			
Social Support	6.07 (3.26)	5.12 (3.21)	5.59 (3.89)
Feedback	4.77 (3.20)	3.70 (2.44)	3.24 (2.08)
Job satisfaction:			
Social Support	5.15 (2.92)	4.84 (2.76)	4.94 (2.93)
Feedback	4.62 (3.67)	3.74 (2.58)	3.06 (2.08)
DCL total score:			
Social Support	57.04 (17.86)	55.56 (19.96)	4.94 (2.93)
Feedback	49.31 (23.25)	44.96 (19.47)	37.76 (14.63) p < 0.01

Moderators

- *Eysenck Personality Questionnaire*: This was only administered at the first assessment occasion. There were no significant differences between the groups on Extroversion, Neuroticism, Psychoticism or Social Conformity.
- *Rosenberg Self-Esteem Scale*: For the Social Support Group scores were 16.30 (3.97), 17.04 (3.97) and 13.89 (3.53). (This represents the scores for the Pre-Intervention phase, the Post-Intervention and Follow-up phases respectively: this format will be used to present all scores for both groups: standard deviations are given in parentheses). Scores for the Feedback Only group were 19.08 (7.83), 16.65 (7.03) and 15.24 (3.88). This group also report improvements in self-esteem, as lower scores on this scale reflect better self-esteem. There were no significant between group differences.
- *Pearlin Mastery Scale*: Scores on this scale for the Social Support Group were 20.41 (3.27), 21.24 (3.68) and 23.11 (3.05). The Feedback

Group scored 21.00 (4.92), 22.09 (4.81) and 22.71 (3.22). Both groups show small improvements in their levels of mastery, but again there are no significant between group differences.

- *The Cooper Coping Skills Scale*: There were no significant differences in coping skills between the groups.
- *The Significant Others Scale*: Actual social support increased over time for the Social Support Group from an average of 4.97 (1.27) to 4.90 (1.09), post-intervention to 5.37 (0.90) at follow-up. The Feedback Group scores were 4.70 (1.21), 4.71 (1.16) and 4.83 (1.12). There were no significant between group differences. Actual practical support also rose over time for both groups. For the Social Support Group scores were 4.64 (1.23), 4.88 (1.02) and 5.09 (1.24). For the Feedback Group scores were 4.65 (1.06), 4.46 (1.05) and 4.76 (0.90). Again while the magnitude of changes is greater for the Social Support groups, there are no significant between group differences.

Stress outcomes

- *General Health Questionnaire*: Both groups show reductions in their levels of psychological distress over time. Scores for the Social Support Group were 3.85 (4.67), 2.60 (3.44) and then finally 2.72 (4.51). For the Feedback Group scores were 5.35 (7.39), 3.17 (6.38) and then 2.53 (4.49). The groups do not differ significantly on any of the test occasions.
- *Maslach Burnout Inventory*: Maslach Emotional Exhaustion scores improved for both groups over time. For the Social Support Group the scores were 20.04 (9.91), 19.80 (8.47) and 19.06 (9.66). For the Feedback Only Group scores were 21.92 (11.39), 19.48 (12.34) and 20.82 (7.66). Depersonalization scores for the Social Support Group were 8.37 (6.45), 8.28 (5.91) and 7.72 (4.46). For the Feedback Group these were 8.96 (6.07), 8.91 (5.38) and 9.65 (4.18). The Social Support Group show a reduction in their level of Depersonalization burnout, whereas the Feedback Only Group show an increase. Finally, both groups show improvements in the Personal Accomplishment scores over time. For the Social Support Group these were 33.52 (7.15), 33.83 (6.47) and then 37.56 (5.98). For the Feedback Group these were 32.46 (7.53), 35.13 (7.55) and 35.59 (6.04).
- *The Minnesota Job Satisfaction Scale*: There were no differences between the groups in satisfaction levels.
- *Sickness Absence*: On average Social Support Group participants took 9.33 (18.17) days off sick in the six months prior to the intervention. By the six-month follow-up, this had reduced to an average of 4.56 days (5.23). For the Feedback Only Group, the respective figures were 10.65 (18.50) and 5.76 (6.83). Again there were no significant between group differences.

Discussion

The results of the Bethlem Maudsley Nursing Stress Intervention Study show that a Social Support-based programme offers no significant advantage over a Feedback Only programme. Why might this be?

Firstly, attendance at Social Support Group sessions was poor. Only three out of 24 participants attended all five sessions. Thirteen attended four sessions. Sometimes staff were unable to attend sessions because of crises on the wards or on account of staffing problems. If staff had been able to receive the full intervention package, the benefits might have been greater. Secondly, while social support is an important moderator of stress, it is clearly only one of a range of such moderators. Carson and Kuipers (1998) have listed at least eight separate moderators, such as personal resilience or hardiness. The current intervention targeted only social support. An intervention that targeted several of these moderators simultaneously would have a better chance of success. Similarly, participants for this study were not selected as having specific problems in the area of social support. It is possible that some, in fact, had good social support networks. Thirdly, stress levels were not excessive in this group of volunteers. The average scores at intake on the General Health Questionnaire were fairly typical of mental health nurses. It would therefore be difficult to see any treatment effect, given that baseline scores were so low. The intake average for the Social Support Group was 3.85, which is below the Caseness score of 5, and well below scores for clinical samples (Carson and Brewerton, 1991). Fourthly, it proved more difficult to recruit participants for the study than was anticipated. Other researchers have reported similar problems with intervention studies with nurses (Kunkler and Whittick, 1991). Similarly the small numbers of participants available for follow-up, 17 in each group, makes it harder to obtain statistically significant changes. The researchers in this study assumed that they would find it easier to recruit participants than proved to be the case.

On a more positive note, there were a number of benefits from the study. For instance, prior to inclusion in the study, participants took on average ten days sickness absence. By the end of the follow-up period, this had reduced to five days. Economically this represents a major saving to the organization. Equally, while the changes in stress and burnout levels were not statistically significant, the trends were all in the right direction. The study led to reductions in stress and burnout levels for those staff who participated in it.

A further study will adopt a multi-method approach to stress reduction, rather than just focusing on social support as in this study. This will be based on the model of Carson and Kuipers (1998) and will involve targeting a range of moderators. Only where a staff member identifies a weakness in a particular area will that area be chosen for intervention. Given the experience of poor attendance with weekly sessions, the new intervention will be delivered via two day workshops. Samples in both groups will also be much larger than in this study.

STUDY 2: THE CLINICAL SUPERVISION EVALUATION PROJECT

Introduction

Despite the importance given to it by almost all professional bodies, there are surprisingly few studies on the effectiveness of clinical supervision. Faugier (1996) confirms this in a review of the field, 'the absence of empirical data on clinical supervision remains widespread in all fields, particularly nursing' (p. 53). Part of the problem no doubt lies with the term 'clinical supervision', which in the eyes of many nurses has a negative managerial connotation. It is only relatively recently that empirical studies into clinical supervision have begun to appear. Hallberg and colleagues at Ersta University College in Sweden have published a series of studies on supervision. The first examined burnout, empathy and sense of coherence amongst district nurses (Palsson et al., 1996). A supervisory group (n = 21) was compared with a comparison group (n = 12) in a quasi-experimental design. The study found no significant effects of supervision on burnout empathy or sense of coherence. The second study, Edberg and Hallberg (1996), found improvements in nurse–patient interactions in an experimental ward with dementia patients, when nurses received training in individualized, planned care and regular, systematic, clinical supervision, compared to a control ward where no changes were made. This is the first-ever study to demonstrate empirically that clinical supervision can directly affect patient care. Finally, a third study with psychiatric nurses (Severinsson and Hallberg, 1996) found that clinical supervision did not affect working milieu or duties, but led to a change in attitudes towards patients and enhanced staffs' sense of personal development.

The Clinical Supervision Evaluation Project is the most systematic attempt to date to investigate empirically the effects of clinical supervision in nursing and health visiting (Butterworth et al., 1996). The study is described in detail elsewhere in this book so the background and methodology will not be covered in depth here. Rather a subsample of the total project sample will be presented to try and answer the question, 'Is clinical supervision good for your mental well-being?'

Butterworth and colleagues were most influenced by the supervision model of Proctor (1986). Proctor has argued that supervision fulfils three main functions which she has labelled normative, formative and restorative. It is difficult to evaluate these components using standardized research tools. For instance, the formative or skills development aspects of clinical supervision are best evaluated through direct observation of skills acquisition *in vivo*. In a study of this magnitude with 23 different research sites, this would clearly have been impossible. Consequently, the measures chosen for the quantitative aspect of the study fit mainly into Proctor's restorative category. The research measures chosen fit into the stress model described earlier (Carson and Kuipers, 1998). Stressors were assessed by the Nurse Stress Index (Harris, 1989). Moderators were measured by a Demographic Checklist and the Cooper Coping Skills Scale. Finally, stress outcomes were assessed by the General Health Questionnaire, the Maslach Burnout Inventory and the Minnesota Job Satisfaction Scale. If clinical supervision is truly good for your mental well-being then we would expect to see reductions in GHQ score, lower Maslach Emotional Exhaustion and increased job satisfaction in nurses and health visitors exposed to clinical supervision.

To answer the question, 'Is clinical supervision good for your mental well-being', we present data below for only two of the groups involved in the Clinical Supervision Evaluation Project. The first group, n = 45, did not receive supervision for the total duration of the project. The second group, n = 90, received clinical supervision throughout the study. Results are presented this way for simplicity.

Results

Only three out of 24 statistical comparisons between the two groups of staff were statistically significant, and two of these occurred at Time 1, before the intervention commenced. Two significant results were obtained for the Minnesota Job Satisfaction Scale. However, as one of these occurred at intake into the study, and did not appear at Time 2, it is difficult to state unequivocally that clinical supervision leads to an increase in job satisfaction. Indeed it is difficult not to escape the conclusion that clinical supervision has no effect on mental well-being.

What might therefore be affecting the mental well-being of nurses and health visitors if it is not clinical supervision? Multiple regression was used with the total project sample (n = 373), for whom complete data were available at the end of 18 months, to see which variables might best predict the three outcome variables discussed in the original stress process model described by Carson and Kuipers (1998). Three variables predicted GHQ Score at Time 3, but only accounted for 13 per cent of the variance. These were alcohol, fitness and Maslach Emotional Exhaustion. So the more someone drinks, the poorer their fitness and the higher their level of Emotional Exhaustion, then the more likely they are to score higher on the GHQ, showing high levels of psychological distress. Maslach Emotional Exhaustion at Time 3 was best predicted by four variables

Table 4.2 Comparison of a group who never received clinical supervision (n = 45) with a group who received clinical supervision throughout the project (n = 90)

	Time 1		Time 2		Time 3	
	No supervision	Supervision	No supervision	Supervision	No supervision	Supervision
Nurse Stress Index	73.63	69.36	68.33	69.84	68.09	70.32
Cooper Coping Skills	114.76	116.87	116.64	118.07	115.95	117.11
Sickness Absence	6.16	7.78	4.36	7.07	15.54	9.02
GHQ Score	5.84	2.85	4.15	3.63	4.02	3.69
		$p < 0.01$				
Minnesota Score	65.62	70.29	66.65	68.91	65.24	68.99
		$p < 0.01$				$p < 0.05$
Maslach Emotional Exhaustion	22.67	19.33	4.96	4.63	4.89	5.24
Maslach Depersonalization	5.93	5.37	4.96	4.63	4.89	5.24
Maslach Personalization Accomplishment	36.40	36.63	35.66	36.83	35.95	35.97

which accounted for 24 per cent of the variance. These were alcohol, Nurse Stress Index Total Score, Maslach Depersonalization and GHQ Total Score. Minnesota Job Satisfaction was affected by three variables which accounted for 13 per cent of the variance. These were age, Nurse Stress Index Total Score and GHQ Total Sore. Mental well-being would therefore appear to be more influenced by variables such as alcohol consumption rather than by clinical supervision. Of course, it is also possible that alcohol use is a consequence rather than a precursor of stress.

Discussion

This sub-analysis of data from the Clinical Supervision Evaluation Project suggests that clinical supervision does not directly affect supervisees' mental well-being. This contradicts the suggestions of other researchers (Everitt *et al.*, 1996; Severinsson and Hallberg, 1996). Why might this be? The first and most obvious possibility is that the measures that we used to evaluate clinical supervision may not have been sensitive enough to change. However, each of the measures has been used in previous research and all have proven reliability and validity. The second possibility is that the nature of the intervention, in this case clinical supervision, may not have been powerful enough to produce change in supervisees. Each of the 23 centres involved in the study delivered clinical supervision in a different format. The researchers simply stipulated a number of essential preconditions, such as not less than 45 minutes to be allocated every four weeks for the process of supervision in the 'active' group. These conditions may not have been stringent enough. Thirdly, the wide variety of specialisms involved may have been a further complication. It may have been better to restrict the study to more homogenous nursing groups focusing on only two specialisms, such as general medical nurses and community mental health nurses. Some nursing specialisms may be more receptive to clinical supervision than others. Fourthly, the authors did not have a satisfactory measure of the supervision process itself. It seems intuitive to suggest that if a supervisee has a good working alliance with his or her supervisor, then this might lead to a better mental health outcome. Conversely, if a supervisee dreads their sessions with their supervisor and sees sessions as punitive in nature, then supervision may have a detrimental effect on their mental health. If we had such a measure available at the commencement of the project, it would have enabled us to have tested the hypothesis that clinical supervision can improve your mental well-being more satisfactorily.

Clearly the Clinical Supervision Evaluation Project has been the most impressive study yet conducted into the effectiveness of clinical supervision. Eighteen-month follow-up data are available on 373 nurses and health visitors. Twenty-three centres in two countries participated in the study. The Project succeeded in its two main aims: to give an informed view on assessment tools, and to report on the activities of selected sites who have evaluated clinical supervision within a specified format. With hindsight some improvements could have been made to the study. It would have been better to have used a randomized controlled design. The addition of a standardized measure of the supervisory process itself would have helped disentangle the effectiveness of supervision. A more focused model of supervision with perhaps fortnightly sessions based on a specific model might also have led to a greater intervention effect. Linked to this, concentration on only two nursing specialisms, instead of the wide variety of specialisms used in the study, might have been more helpful.

STRESS MANAGEMENT, CLINICAL SUPERVISION AND SOCIAL SUPPORT

Both interventions described in this chapter, a social support training package and clinical supervision, were designed to try to reduce nursing staff stress. Neither was wholly successful in achieving this aim. What lessons can we learn from these studies with respect to stress management interventions in nursing?

Long (1998) describes the Swindon Staff Support Service Model, which locates the above interventions within a much broader staff support strategy. The Swindon model incorporates the following components:

- Personal development training: This includes training in counselling skills, how to break bad news, how to handle verbal aggression and bullying, and how to deal with loss, grief and bereavement. Workshops are also provided for staff in time management and assertion skills.
- Counselling and psychotherapy: A range of therapeutic approaches is available to staff who want access to counselling or psychotherapy with professionally accredited therapists.
- Professional support: Support sessions are provided for managers and isolated professionals to be able to discuss work-related or personal difficulties confidentially with a member of the Staff Support Service. These sessions are not as regular as counselling sessions.
- Meditation and relaxation groups.
- Personal stress care programmes: These are offered to a small number of staff on long-term sick leave. An initial assessment by the Staff Support Service is followed by an intensive programme based on an holistic mind, body and spirit approach.
- Complementary therapies: Staff are allowed access to subsidized aromatherapy, yoga, shiatsu and reflexology.

There are, however, methodological problems in applying stress management approaches to nursing staff. In two key critical papers, Briner and Reynolds (1993) and Reynolds and Briner (1994), the authors suggest that:

'occupational stress reduction ... is one of the many fads initiated by academics, commercialised by consultants and embraced by managers but that ultimately fail to deliver the panacea-like solutions which they promise.' (Reynolds and Briner, 1994, p. 75)

They point out that most of the employees entering into stress management workshops may not be suffering from clinical levels of distress. For instance, while the 'caseness' rate for the GHQ-28 is set at a score of 5 or more, the average score for clinical samples is 10 (Carson and Brewerton, 1991). While there has been a great deal of concern over the issues of staff stress and burnout, the actual incidence of burnout and stress may be lower than many researchers would have us believe. If we adopt a strict definition of burnout, that is the individual has to score high on Emotional Exhaustion, high on Depersonalization and low on Personal Accomplishment on the Maslach Scale, then we find that only around 5 per cent of ward-based mental health nurses meet this strict criterion (Fagin *et al.*, 1996). Interventions should be targeted at this group, rather than being offered to all staff whether they require them or not.

There is also a danger of locating the problem of stress within the individual nurse, who is said not to be able to cope with the pressure of work. Such a perspective ignores the contribution of the organization, and indeed government, in contributing to stress at work. Bruggen (1997) has recently provided a comprehensive account of the effects of organizational changes on National Health Service staff.

CONCLUSIONS

Clinical supervision is essential in ensuring that nurses and other professionals practise in a responsible and reflective manner (Bishop, 1998). However, its effects are clearly complex. Supervision may work in different ways for the participants receiving it. The Clinical Supervision Evaluation Project focused largely on the restorative aspects of clinical supervision, which did not seem to alter much over an 18-month period. Normative and formative aspects of the supervision process were much harder to measure. It could be argued that organizations offering clinical supervision to all staff, regardless of perceived need, may have little research evidence on which to justify this provision. In fairness, it should be remembered that clinical supervision is not a panacea. Indeed, some might argue why should clinical supervision work, given the huge range of other factors that impinge on the working lives of nurses, and which may have a greater bearing on staffs' emotional well-being. Similarly, do we have the research tools to adequately capture the dynamic nature of the supervision process, which is insufficiently measured in pre- and post-tests. At this stage in the evolution of our knowledge, clinical supervision may be more driven by policy imperatives than by evidence of its direct benefit to staff or organizations. Its effects on the nature of the nurse–patient relationships are even harder to evaluate. Future research into clinical supervision needs to be grounded better in theory, and more tightly controlled experimentally, so we are better able to discern its effects.

ACKNOWLEDGEMENTS

The contribution of Professor Veronica Bishop to the setting up and design of the Clinical Supervision Evaluation Project is warmly recognized. Professor Ted White, Julie Jeacock and April Clements were key members of the core research team, and their support was critical in carrying out the research. The Project was funded by the Department of Health for England and Wales and by the Scottish Home and Health Department. The Bethlem Maudsley Nursing Stress Intervention Study was funded by the Trust's Health Services Research Group. The contributions of the following colleagues is appreciated: Professor Kevin Gournay, Professor Julian Leff, Professor Elizabeth Kuipers, Dr Frank Holloway, Ben Thomas, Maria West and Sukwinder Maal. The social support groups were facilitated by Jane Bunclark and Joanne Cavagin.

REFERENCES

Bishop, V. (1998) *Clinical Supervision in Practice: Some Questions, Answers and Guidelines*, Macmillan/NT Research, London.

Bowling, A. (1995) *Measuring Disease*, Open University Press, Buckingham, UK.

Briner, R. and Reynolds, S. (1993) Bad theory and bad practice in occupational stress, *The Occupational Psychologist*, **19**, 8–13.

Bruggen, P. (1997) *Who Cares? True Stories of the NHS Reforms*, Jon Carpenter, Charlbury, UK.

Butterworth, A., Bishop, V. and Carson, J. (1996) First steps towards evaluating clinical supervision in nursing and health visiting. Part 1: Theory, policy and practice development: A review, *Journal of Clinical Nursing*, **5**(1), 25–35.

Carson, J. and Brewerton, T. (1991) Out of the clinic into the classroom, *Adults Learning*, **2**(9), 256–7.

Carson, J. and Kuipers, E. (1998) Stress management interventions, in Hardy, S., Carson, J. and Thomas, B. (eds) *Occupational Stress: Personal and Professional Approaches*, Stanley Thornes, Cheltenham.

Cooper, C., Sloan, S. and Williams, S. (1998) *Occupational Stress Indicator Management Guide*, NFER-Nelson, Windsor, UK.

Cronin-Stubbs, D. and Brophy, E. (1985) Burnout: Can social support save the psychiatric nurse?' *Journal of Psycho-social Nursing*, **23**(7), 8–13.

Dawkins, J., Depp, F. and Selzer, N. (1985) Stress and the psychiatric nurse, *Journal of Psycho-social Nursing*, **23**(11), 9–15.

Edberg, A. and Hallberg, I. (1996) Effects of clinical supervision on nurse–patient interaction quality: A controlled study in dementia care, *Clinical Nursing Research*, **5**(1), 127–49.

Everitt, J., Bradshaw, T. and Butterworth, T. (1996) Stress and clinical supervision in mental health care, *Nursing Times*, **92**(1), 34–5.

Eysenck, H. and Eysenck, S. (1991) *Manual of the Eysenck Personality Scales (EPS Adult)*, Hodder & Stoughton, London.

Fagin, L., Carson, J., Leary, J., DeVilliers, N., Bartlett, H., O'Malley, P., West, M., McElfatrick, S. and Brown, D. (1996) Stress, coping and burnout in mental health nurses: Findings from three research studies, *The International Journal of Social Psychiatry*, **42**(1), 102–11.

Faugier, J. (1996) Clinical supervision in mental health nursing, in Sandford, T. and Gourney, K. (eds), *Perspectives in Mental Health Nursing*, Ballière Tindall, London.

Goldberg, D. and Williams, P. (1988) *A User's Guide to the General Health Questionnaire*, NFER-Nelson, Windsor, UK.

Grey-Toft, P. and Anderson, J. (1981) The Nursing Stress Scale: Development of an instrument, *Journal of Behavioural Assessment*, **3**, 11–23.

Harris, P. (1989) The Nurse Stress Index, *Work and Stress*, **5**(4), 335–46.

Hipwell, A., Tyler, P. and Wilson, C. (1989) Sources of stress and dissatisfaction among nurses in four hospital environments, *British Journal of Medical Psychology*, **62**, 71–9.

Kunkler, J. and Whittick, J. (1991) Stress management groups for nurses: Practical problems and possible solutions, *Journal of Advanced Nursing*, **16**, 172–6.

Long, J. (1998) Providing support systems for health care staff, in Hardy, S., Carson, J. and Thomas, B. (eds) (1998) op. cit.

Love, C. and Hunter, M. (1996) Violence in public sector psychiatric hospitals: Benchmarking nursing staff injury rates, *Journal of Psychosocial Nursing*, **34**(5), 30–4.

Maslach, C. and Jackson, S. (1986) *Maslach Burnout Inventory*, Consulting Psychologists Press, California.

Norbeck, J. (1985) Types and sources of social support for managing job stress in critical care nursing, *Nursing Research*, **30**, 225–30.

Palsson, M., Hallberg, I., Norberg, A. and Bjorvell, H. (1996) Burnout, empathy and sense of coherence among Swedish district nurses before and after systematic clinical supervision, *Scandinavian Journal of Caring Science*, **10**(1), 19–26.

Pearlin, L. and Schooler, C. (1978) The structure of coping, *Journal of Health and Social Behaviour*, **19**, 2–21.

Pierce, G., Lakey, B., Sarason, I. and Sarason, B. (1997) *Sourcebook of Social Support and Personality*, Plenum, New York.

Power, M., Champion, L. and Aris, S. (1988) The development of a measure of social support: The Significant Others (SOS) Scale, *British Journal of Clinical Psychology*, **27**, 348–58.

Proctor, B. (1986) Supervision: A co-operative exercise in accountability, in Marken M. and Payne, M. (eds) *Enabling and Ensuring: Supervision in Practice*, National Youth Bureau and Council for Education and Training in Youth and Community Work, Leicester, UK.

Proudfoot, J., Guest, D., Carson, J., Dunn, G. and Gray, J. (1997) Effects of cognitive-behavioural training in job finding among long-term unemployed people, *The Lancet*, **350**, 96–100.

Reynolds, S. and Briner, R. (1994) Stress management at work: With whom, for whom, and to what ends? *British Journal of Guidance and Counselling*, **22**(1), 75–89.

Ritter, S., Tolchard, B. and Stewart, R. (1995) Coping with stress in mental health nursing, in Carson, J., Fagin, L. and Ritter, S. (eds) *Stress and Coping in Mental Health Nursing*, Chapman & Hall, London.

Rosenberg, M. (1965) *Society and the Adolescent Self-Image*, Princeton University Press, Princeton.

Severinsson, E. and Hallberg, I. (1996) Systematical clinical supervision, working milieu and influence over duties: The psychiatric nurses' viewpoint. A pilot study. *International Journal of Nursing Studies*, **33**(4), 394–406.

Weiss, D., Dawis, R., England, G. and Lofquist, L. (1967) *Manual for the Minnesota Satisfaction Questionnaire*, University of Minnesota Industrial Relations Centre, Minnesota.

Wheeler, H. (1997) A review of occupational stress research, *British Journal of Nursing*, **6**(11), 642–5.

Wycherley, B. (1987) *The Living Skills Pack*, South East Thames Regional Health Authority, Bexhill, UK.

Yalom, D. (1985) *The Theory and Practice of Group Psychotherapy*, Basic Books, New York.

5 | Psychiatric nursing

Phil Barker

'While she was away I thought she must be a very new nurse: she had not yet become inhuman, but was trying to learn the trick.'

(Welch, 1983)

ARMING OURSELVES

People who think they know what is best for others should not be taken too seriously. Indeed, as some have suggested, such people may even be dangerous (Rowe, 1989). Any consideration of psychiatric nursing, its practice and its value must, therefore, accommodate the unknown as a balance for what little knowledge we do possess.

It is commonly accepted that quality psychiatric nursing involves the 'therapeutic use of self'. Some North American nurses have long argued that this activity, or rather its expression through interpersonal relationships, is the very basis of psychiatric nursing (Peplau, 1986). Travelbee (1971) has noted, for example, that nursing 'is an interpersonal process because it is always concerned with people either directly or indirectly'. This principle is clearly relevant, however, to just about every other caring group. Butterworth (1987) has declared the patent need for psychiatric nurses in the UK to demonstrate expertise in interpersonal relationships and therapeutic use of self, suggesting that the fine detail of such activity might in some way distinguish the ideology of psychiatric nursing. The long pedigree of interpersonal relationship building skills and theory possessed by North American nurses is beyond challenge (Schwartz and Shockley, 1956). It is not yet clear, however, whether British nurses' current interest in the same territory represents an equivalent ideology, science of ideas, or reflection of a consistent theoretical rationale (Altschul, 1972). It can be accepted as a canon of faith that the nurse's manipulation of her/himself, during contact with the person who is the patient, characterizes psychiatric nursing practice. It is less easy to believe, however, that nurses, or the people in their care, always understand what exactly is taking place.

The significance of what exactly is meant by 'self' and therefore its therapeutic use is critical to the area of supervision in psychiatric nursing. It is an unsafe assumption that any psychiatric nurse possesses only one 'self' which is manipulated to positive effect with a wide range of people in care across a range of situations.

I suspect that nurses often use 'themselves' as a subtle controlling, manipulative force, in an effort to change the people in their care, somehow 'for the better'. This is not only characteristic of nurses, but of all carers, professional or lay, who are inclined to feel guilty when 'not doing enough'. The therapeutic use of self can be benign and kindly, or it can be openly challenging and confrontational. Some would argue that the attempt to make people conform, whether subtle or gross, is an outstanding characteristic of all psychotherapies (Masson, 1989). Hence the current concern for the emotional security of all who might be offered help which involves the professional's 'therapeutic use of self'.

DISARMING

Supervision in psychiatric nursing has two main aims: to protect people in care from nurses and to protect nurses from themselves. In dealing with the protection of people in care I do not wish to address issues involving the overt, intentional, abuse of people in care, although I am aware that examples of malpractice continue to be reported. Rather, I wish to focus on situations where people in care receive unnecessary or over-zealous direction from nurses who believe that they know what is 'best'. Given my belief that nurses should be involved in 'empowering' people in care, this might be termed a problem of benign paternalism. Psychiatric medicine, like its mainstream equivalent, involves the treatment of people with mental disorder, with or without their consent. Psychiatric nursing may manipulate aspects of the person's 'illness' as part of care, but is not concerned directly with treatment. Nursing manipulates the person's relationship with illness.

THE HELPING RELATIONSHIP

A distinction needs to be made here between the related concepts of 'helpfulness' and 'helping'. Nurses are portrayed, traditionally, as professionals who try to be helpful. Invariably this means that they intervene on behalf of the person in care. Nurses who guide a person away from danger in the direction of safety are, quite reasonably, seen to be helpful. Preventing a person from harming him or herself, or others, is a helpful action. Calming people who are anxious and frightened, raising the spirits of those who are in despair can all be seen as helpful. Such actions, however, have little to do with the promotion of growth and development. Indeed, dependency in its various forms can be traced directly to the helpful actions of nurses and others. Clearly, nurses need to 'be helpful' in their everyday work with people in care. Such helpful actions are part and parcel of any social system in which interdependence is the rule and genuine independence is rare. Helpfulness is the support system which characterizes all social units. It is, therefore, an integral part of nursing. In my view it is not the most important part of nursing. We should not lose sight of the fact, however, that the more useful we are, the more useless the person might become.

Helping is about arranging ways of promoting growth and development. Often, such actions begin with something akin to 'being helpful', but thereafter the controlling emphasis moves gradually from the nurse to the person in care. People can experience sudden waves of emotion which precipitate aggressive acts, panic–flight–fright behaviour, or may 'paralyse' them. Highlighting the significant events or the person's thoughts or beliefs about the situation may 'be helpful' in clarifying the experience for the person. The nurse may be able to use such information as a basis for developing some alternative way of responding to, or dealing with, such situations. This may also be seen as 'helpful'. The challenge for the nurse lies in being able to transfer her part in this interpretation, clarification, resolution to the person in care. If she fails to do this, the person will become dependent upon her as a means of resolving her emotional problems.

THE MEANING OF LIFE

The psychological or psychiatric problems discussed above represent, in my view, problems of living. Although we are emphasizing here 'mental' problems, the difficulties experienced by people with long-term physical illnesses or disabilities would be similar. Living with an amputation, unstable diabetes or a memory defect following head injury creates enormous problems of everyday living. Nurses, and other health-care professionals, are often tempted to express understanding of the disability: 'We know how you feel'. Helping a person identify, confront, overcome or otherwise manage a life problem requires our awareness of what such a problem might mean for us. The care of older people, which has at least in recent years been characterized by appalling standards of care, serves as a good example of the problem we face in pursuing true understanding of the person's problems of living.

Although it would be convenient for us to believe that some older people experience a 'second childhood', this is hardly correct. From middle age onwards our mastery of our bodies, our emotions and of reality is reversed. Life is, for all of us, an onward march to the grave: there is no going back, except in our imagination. Older people can be, indeed often are, treated like children, when their faculties begin to fail them. Such care fails to acknowledge what the experience of ageing and diminishing capability might mean to the older person. We need to consider whether or not such 'care' is a reflection of our own inadequacy in dealing with the inevitability of decay and death.

Understanding, which is at the heart of all care, may be hard to come by, especially where the young and beautiful are forced to confront the transitory nature of their suppleness and good looks.

Physical empathy involves our 'understanding' of the vulnerability which we share with the afflicted person in our care. Where physical pathology is concerned we often console ourselves with the notion that our chance of being similarly affected is either remote or that an effective remedy would be available. Young people probably still pretend, as my own generation did, that they hope they'll die before they get old.

Psychological empathy is more intimidating. It involves our understanding of the emotional experience of the person. Here too, the nurse identifies strongly with the person, who unwittingly holds up a mirror to his carer. Often the reflection is too hard to bear; the background awareness that there is no panacea for emotional suffering, that psychological distress often simply has to run its course, can be borne easily only by the stoical or the wise. The easiest options are to deny the experience in ourselves, or to diminish the importance of the experience for the person. Given the psychological threat involved in empathic relationships, it is little wonder that people in care often feel that few really understand them. When the nurse says 'I know how you feel', she may merely be mouthing a worthless cliché or dealing with a mere hypothesis.

'This is how I would feel if I were in your shoes: thankfully I'm not!' This is a fragile kind of understanding. To be empathic we need to focus all our attention on the person's description of his experience. Ironically, we might appear to possess more understanding if we professed it less. Goffman (1968) described the manipulation of the patient [sic] as 'degradation therapy', whereby he was obliged to take on the staff's version of himself as a necessary condition of treatment. Manipulation is also possible in a more benign form whenever carers exercise a belief that they know 'what is happening within the person'. Although some people in care may find it difficult to describe their experiences, carers need to question what is to be gained by advocating that they accept our construction of their reality. Holding back from making such interpretations can be immensely difficult, especially where nurses assume that such interpretations are at the very heart of psychiatric practice. Helping nurses to consider how they view and respond to the person's experience is one of the supervisor's tasks.

The special characteristic of psychiatric nursing involves the nurse's 'use of self' in the medium of the helping process. Although, as noted earlier, psychiatric nurses can also provide 'helpful', short-term interventions, the nature of such 'helpful' actions and the process by which they can be developed (preceptorship) does not differ significantly from other branches of nursing. 'Learning the ropes' involves the supervisor asking the question 'How can I help you meet this standard?' The truly special demands of psychiatric nursing require the supervisor to ask a much more fundamental question. The supervisor *needs* to establish that the nurse knows what the patient's *needs* are, so that she might establish 'what *needs* to be done'. Having discussed the presentation of the patient at any particular point in time, the supervisor might ask: 'What is it that you need to do?' (Keith-Lucas, 1972). From this base grows a range of questions which increase in complexity the simpler they become:

- What are your reasons for choosing *that*?
- What are your alternatives?
- How do you know you can do that?
- What do you think will happen?
- How will you decide?
- What do you need me for?'

The supervisor is not in a position of determining what needs to be done, although this may be very clear in her own mind. Rather, she is concerned to establish whether or not the novice is clear about her objectives and, more importantly, is willing to do what needs to be done. Given the emphasis upon interpersonal relationships, psychiatric nursing is a potential emotional minefield. Supervision is largely about helping the nurse to know what her choices are and to decide whether or not she is ready to take them.

THE FOCUS ON THE PERSON

The focus on the person in care, the process of caring for him or her, and the acknowledgement of the nurse's needs, are intertwined. For the purpose of clarifying each of these I shall deal with them separately. Issues concerning the nurse's relationship with the person begin with their first meeting and end, literally, when last they meet. This relationship is, therefore, the ground upon which the care plan is laid, running the very length of their encounter. The stages involved in identifying and clarifying the person's needs, trying to meet them and evaluating their outcome can be distinguished as units of the care plan. This distinction is, however artificial since needs are more likely to be stated, re-stated and adapted throughout the helping encounter, as are the means of helping deployed by the nurse. Psychiatric nursing, if it is to be anything, should be an organic process. The nurse's helping should be integrated fully with the needs and nature of the person in care, in the same way as a plant coexists with the soil from which it gains its sustenance and support. The supervisor needs to be aware of the organic nature of the care process under review: the supervisory process needs to be similarly reflexive and diffuse.

Despite this diffuse nature there clearly exists a need for structure upon which to base the supervisory process. In reality, the nurse's relationship with the person in care will ebb and flow, from involvement in discrete goal-orientated activities to contemplation and reflection. The nurse's experience of caring will change in a similar fashion: at times she will be more aware of herself than of the person; at others the 'activity' will override them both. It may be helpful to begin by examining these different relationships.

The relationships

Given the assumed interpersonal basis of psychiatric nursing, attention needs to be paid to the interaction of nurse and 'patient'. The founding father of the 'interpersonal school' of psychiatry, Harry Stack Sullivan, saw all psychiatry as:

'*the study of processes that involve or go on between people. The field of interpersonal relations, under any and all circumstances in which these relations exist ... a personality can never be isolated from the complex of interpersonal relations in which the person lives and has his being.*'(Sullivan, 1947, p. 4)

It may be most expedient to look at the relationship from the nurse's viewpoint, since she is the 'reporter'. The supervisor should not lose sight of the fact that the relationship is reciprocal, and the nurse may need to extend her 'experience' in an attempt to embrace the person's view of the care he (or she) receives and of his carer.

Four main relationships need to be examined. For reasons which are practical and logical we shall begin with the relationship which is furthest removed from the person in care. The nurse's relationship with her supervisor will be discussed first, since this is the primary relationship: the one which is happening in the 'here-and-now'. The nurse's relationship with the care plan will be considered next; followed by the nurse's relationship with herself, in terms of her 'use of self' in the caring process, and her personal reactions (reflections) on caring. The relationship with the person in care will be considered last since this was the starting point and is, therefore, furthest from the supervisory relationship currently operating.

1. Nurse and supervisor

Supervision which is not built upon an open, trusting, positive relationship will be virtually useless. Allocated supervisors should be aware of what, exactly, they are offering: is this an equal or a hierarchical relationship? The former will encourage exploration, discovery and growth; the latter will achieve more limited goals and may even foster dependency, or resentment. The supervisor–protégé relationship must begin with an examination of the underlying philosophy:

- Why are we meeting?
- What are our aims?
- What do we believe is important?

Once this is clarified, attention can turn to how the relationship might 'work'. If the nurse has not expressly selected her guide and mentor, then he or she needs to clarify what might be the limits of this supervisory relationship (or the limitations of his/her supervisor).

It has been noted earlier that the supervisor–protégé relationship reflects the clinical caring relationship. Both aim for growth and development, acceptance or adjustment. Practical details, such as how often sessions last, how often they take place, who defines the agenda and keeps the notes, etc., can be arranged with ease, possibly at the first meeting. Ritter (1989) provides detailed guidelines, comprising 23 'actions' with supporting rationales, which define the practical process of supervision. Arranging means of communicating 'needs', expressing feelings, discussing 'taboo' topics, or simply exposing oneself to another may take much longer. Psychiatric problems are akin to icebergs. What do I do if I fear that the person I am working with at present is planning to kill himself. Do I tell my 'new' supervisor now, or do I simply review the 'tip' which is visible? The answer reveals the extent to which I trust my supervisor, if not also myself. The supervisor must not only demonstrate that she (or he) is trustworthy, but also that she can help the nurse trust herself.

How does such a relationship develop? This is a question similar to 'how long is a piece of string?' My experience suggests that every supervisory relationship is different, since the pairings are different. What is common to them all is the need to maintain monitoring – a watching brief. Supervisor and protégé make a commitment when first they meet. This commits both parties to a policy of frankness, discipline and a mutual concern for the welfare of the person in care. Both parties need to review, at appropriate intervals, the development of their working relationship, checking on its healthiness and the general state of play. All relationships are characterized by three elements:

- *congruence*, where both parties relate to one another on the basis of largely realistic pictures of themselves and each other;
- *collusion*, where both tacitly agree not to notice largely inaccurate self-conceptions in one or both of them;
- *contest*, where one or both of them try to impose their definitions of themselves, or the other, on the other person.

Clearly, the hierarchical preceptor role described above reinforces contest, since the supervisor defines herself as the 'knowing' and the nurse as the 'ignorant'. Since this form of supervision is engineered, usually as part of an operational policy, there may also be a requirement for collusion. This is most likely where the 'learned' status of the supervisor is not readily apparent, but for organizational reasons must not be acknowledged.

Supervisors who are congruent will be the most successful and satisfying. Often this will involve them in losing themselves (i.e. temporarily turning away from their own values and personal concerns) by getting involved with the concerns of the protégé. Losing oneself in this manner projects an unconditional acceptance of the protege (warts and all), and a willingness to share empathically her experience of care.

2. Nurse and care plan

The supervisory process must include a critical appraisal of the care currently provided, with a view to amending or supplementing this, or changing direction completely. Although 'intellectual' in character, this examination involves the nurse's relationship with her work, which is an extension of herself. By its very nature this examination is potentially threatening and may raise issues and anxieties which will need to be addressed in the next part of the 'relationship'.

The supervisor encourages the nurse to assess the care plan at both a 'global' level, and in fine detail. In my experience the critical features of all care plans are similar, irrespective of the setting in which care is conducted, or the population involved. In Figure 5.1 these core features are illustrated in the form used by my colleagues in an intensive psychiatric care setting (Barker *et al.*, 1997). This format serves as the skeleton for the nurse's discussion with her supervisor. Each aspect of the care plan is discussed and rated, in terms of its relative value and comments are made as appropriate. The aspects considered include:

- the 'working relationship' with the person in care or significant others;
- her ability to organize the various stages of the care plan;

- her ability to identify and resolve problems met at any stage;
- her use and understanding of the various technical aspects of care.

Given that nurse's reports on progress and incidental events are so important, these are included in the supervisory review.

The supervisor invites the nurse to describe the care plan to date, explaining what has been done and why. In addition to this 'subjective' evaluation by the nurse herself, the supervisor may also ask to see materials connected with the care plan, for example completed assessment charts, visual aids or record forms designed for use by staff or the person himself, diaries, notes, graphs and other summary charts, as well as progress notes. The supervisor may consider it appropriate to sample the care process more directly by 'sitting in' on selected sessions, providing that this is agreeable to both the nurse and the person himself. Alternatively, the supervisor may ask the nurse to record or tape sample interactions, with the same ethical proviso, to add a further dimension to the profile of the care process.

Some supervisors advocate making discrete judgements, in the form of ratings, of the various elements involved in the care plan (Barker, 1987). Ideally, both nurse and supervisor should use the same format to compare notes on their interpretation of the elements comprising Figure 5.1, comparing their ratings and associated comments afterwards. Such a procedure encourages critical self-examination (from the nurse's perspective), whilst encouraging supervisors to be specific about perceived assets and deficits within the overall care plan. My experience suggests that emphasis upon the supervisor's 'objective' evaluation of the care plan can be transferred gradually to the nurse's subjective assessment of her own work. The supervisor's feedback helps the nurse reinforce her awareness of specific areas of competence or deficiency. The nurse is given an opportunity to look at her work initially through her supervisor's eyes, as a stepping stone towards a more objective self-examination (if that is not a contradiction in terms).

Although all aspects of the care plan are important, some elements might be seen as more vital than others. Supervisors may wish to focus more attention on areas such as confidentiality, ethical issues, the management of medication and other medical treatments, such as ECT, the person's role in the care plan (consent), and problems involving the safety of the person, other patients or the nurse's colleagues.

3. Nurse and self

The nurse's relationship with herself focuses mainly upon her expectations of what she should be doing, or her view of what she has already done. This appraisal considers what demands the care setting makes of the

CLINICAL SUPERVISION RECORD

Name:_____

A: General	Rating	Comments
1. Relationship with person 2. Relationship with significant others 3. Organization of care plan 4. Problem-solving		
B: Assessment		
1. Selection of method 2. Handling of method 3. Use of guidelines 4. Rationale 5. Patient orientation 6. Patient expectation		
C: Plan		
1. Problems/strengths 2. Goals 3. Nursing action 4. Rationale 5. Intervention methods 6. Evaluation method		
D: Progress		
1. Organization of evaluation 2. Implementation of evaluation 3. Adaptation and modification		
E: Reporting		
1. Content 2. Style 3. Presentation		

Supervisor   Date   Nurse   Date

_____   _____   _____   _____

Figure 5.1 Clinical supervision record used in an intensive psychiatric care setting (Barker *et al.*, 1997)

nurse. This can range from concerns about her work environment, workload, shift systems, noise, irregularities in circadian rhythms, demands on sleep–wakefulness, and so on, all of which can be stressful. The nurse needs an opportunity to review, comment, even simply to complain about coping with these pressures. In some cases the supervisor might consider it appropriate to encourage the nurse to suggest and experiment with possible 'solutions' using a negotiated timescale.

Consideration is also given to the demands she makes of herself. Some nurses find it difficult to cope with changes which they are required to make 'within themselves' in order to fulfil the person's needs. In others, the very nature of decision-making and taking responsibility for specific individuals, acting as a primary nurse or keyworker, will bring their own pressures. Her 'failure' to respond to these demands may prove emotionally distressing. It is one of the supervisor's tasks to determine whether the source of any stress lies within the organization, or within the individual nurse (Hare *et al.*, 1988). Unnecessary environmental stresses can be removed or reduced. Poor work rotas, inadequate equipment, lack of physical and moral support, all can be 'fixed', with a resultant reduction of stress. Where the stress lies in the nurse's 'use of self', the adjustment must be made on a personal level.

In psychiatric care much attention needs to be paid to the nurse's personal expectations. If she believes she should be able to help everyone towards successful rehabilitation or 'full growth', failure to achieve such lofty aims will be distressing. Where she is working with people who try to kill themselves, who reject her help, or who are dying or deteriorating from some physical cause (as with confused older people), her inability to help may generate strong feelings of guilt (Carder and Hall, 1981). Negative emotions which are experienced in such situations need to be acknowledged openly (Pryser, 1984). Although this appraisal ties in closely with the analysis of care goals and outcome mentioned above, specific attention needs to be paid here to the nurse's beliefs and feelings about 'cure' and 'rehabilitation'. What does she think is a 'good result'? The supervisor should be aware that 'psychic stress' is more likely where the person in care is regressed, aggressive, unmotivated, dependent, resistive or in some way 'incurable' (Vanderpool, 1984).

Care needs to be taken not to add to the nurse's difficulties by being too confrontational. The supervisor should be aware of the risk that the nurse might disguise or deny her fears and anxieties, or stifle feelings of frustration, interpreting these as signs of her own failure (Parkes, 1972). She may fear admitting such failings to her supervisor, especially if she appears to be a 'masterly' practitioner. The supervisor may need to model her own 'human frailty', by disclosing examples of her own fears, anxieties and frustrations, drawn from her own clinical experience. (From this perspective, supervision of one clinical nurse by another practitioner is almost essential.) The need to use disclosure, to facilitate sharing of common negative feelings, may be greatest in care of people with chronic mental disorder (Firth *et al.*, 1987; Jones *et al.*, 1987) or severe dementia (Athlin and Norberg, 1987). In either of these cases the nurse might feel that she should only experience positive feelings towards such 'unfortunates'. Her very real experiences of anger, frustration (or even fear and loathing of certain individuals) will generate extreme guilt. If properly accessed, clarified and discussed, the nurse may be able to accept such feelings as a natural part of the experience of caring.

4. Nurse and person in care

The nurse's relationship with the person in care must emphasize 'personal' characteristics over 'clinical' considerations. If the nurse is inexperienced and apprehensive about the supervisory process, fairly focused questioning might enable her to begin framing a picture of what has happened so far in this relationship, as a basis for drawing upon her more subjective feelings: 'How often have you seen him (or her)? Where do you meet? For how long? What have you discussed?' These pointed enquiries lead to more open-ended, general questions designed to allow the nurse more freedom to choose both the content focus and the emphasis she wishes to give. This 'wide-angle' focus is the starting point for the nurse with more experience of supervision. Typical opening questions might include:

'So how did you find Mr J ...?' (inviting direct observation)
'How do you think your work with Mr J . . . is going?' (inviting intellectual reflection)
'How do you feel about this man?' (inviting emotional reflection)
'How do you think he feels about you, so far?' (inviting empathic statement).

This relationship underpins the three relationships already discussed. All of them are involved in a kind of dance. The nurse tries to identify the direction in which the person is moving: What needs is he pursuing? Where is he going? She tries to follow him, responding to things he says or does, sometimes in an attempt to be 'helpful', at others to 'help' him progress further in the required direction. Her actions will often prompt certain responses, encouraging him to do things, embrace certain ideas or even try to manipulate certain emotions. Supervision focuses upon what exactly is happening in this relationship. If, for example, the person describes himself as 'depressed', this description is not so much a statement of a natural emotion, as the application of a technical label, previously 'learned' by the person. The nurse needs to establish early on what this means. The person might then describe feelings of 'hopelessness', which in turn breed despair, lethargy and thoughts of suicide. The nurse's response to these sentiments has a major bearing on the developing relationship. Does she challenge this 'defeatist' talk, or does she encourage further exploration and reflection? The nurse who tries to draw the person 'back to reality' (as she understands it) too quickly might simply advance the retreat being undertaken. Alternatively, the nurse who facilitates further discussion of these feelings, might serve as a prop, encouraging forward movement on the part of the person. The supervisor's role is to help the nurse to clarify how she sees the person, and to consider what he might see in her. At the same time consideration of the relationship triad – congruence, collusion and contest – might help her appreciate not only what is happening, but also what needs to be done.

CONCLUSION

Supervision is now established as a critical component in determining, at least, the security of staff in monitoring their work and in managing their potential occupational stress. In time it should become clearer to what extent the supervisory process increases our chances of ensuring that 'quality' care is offered to everyone, and that as few nurses as possible suffer in the process. Nursing is beginning to become more business-like. Those who manage services want to be able to measure the quality of care and want to know that financial cost is translated into effective care. This chapter has focused attention upon some of the issues which have been central to the art and science of psychiatric nursing over almost 50 years. It is relatively easy to define and establish 'procedures' which are part and parcel of institutional life (see Ritter, 1989, for an excellent example). It is easy to operationalize the process for delivering anxiolytic medication. But what is the most 'effective' procedure for assessing whether this measure is necessary, how it will be received, and judging the alternatives? I am confident, also, in the belief that it is less easy to operationalize 'procedures' which might help people to feel valued, to confront their deeper anxieties, to live in the 'real world', or to share their lives with others. Organic nursing, like organic gardening, is a dirty business, and some people simply can't stand the smell.

It is reassuring to see the appearance of a second edition of this book. This means that clinical supervision and mentorship are not passing fads, but have been embedded into the culture of nursing. Supervision is, however, like hearing a welcome voice when lost in the dark. We are reassured, for the moment, but we know we can still become lost here, or somewhere else, again in the dark future. But still the reassurance is warmly accepted. Psychiatric nurses, at any stage of their professional development, are potentially vulnerable creatures. If they are to shed their professional uniformed cover and 'get involved' with the people in their care at a human level, they risk exposing all their own human frailties and foibles. This may be too hot for some to handle. Effective clinical supervision can help turn down the heat, or help us acclimatize better.

I have already seen supervision grow within my own ambit of practice. Currently, in my clinical role, I have experience of at least three kinds of supervision. I supervise individual nurse clinicians; I facilitate group supervision; and I am a member of a peer-supervision group. The latter is, for me, the most challenging and exciting. Although the group of clinicians who meet every week range from a first-year staff to myself (the Professor) with 30 years experience, we all meet on the same plane of experience; and work towards sharing those experiences equally. It is very uplifting to receive support as well as 'challenges' from colleagues who are not only so much younger, but also who (traditionally) would be seen as less experienced. We have found that all our experiences are 'different' but valuable.

We need to explore many different kinds of supervisory format if we are to avoid allowing some nurses to 'burn out' through over-committment, or to continue to hide behind professional masks which people in care will, like Denton Welch, find unpleasantly unhelpful. Supervision, providing that it is properly handled, might be the salvation of both the nurse and the person in care. The thread which I have tried to draw through this chapter represents a concern for welfare: the best interests of the person in care and of his/her carer. Hence my concern to protect people in care from nurses and nurses from themselves. Without supervision the 'quality nurse' will sacrifice herself for the best interests of her 'patient' – she will burn out. With supervision, we can have some guarantee of quality care without the risk of emotional life and limb.

REFERENCES

Altschul, A. T. (1972) *Patient–Nurse Interaction: A Study of Interactive Patterns on Acute Psychiatric Wards*, Churchill Livingstone, Edinburgh.

Athlin, E. and Norberg, A. (1987) Caregivers' attitudes to and interpretations of the behaviour of severely demented patients during feeding in a patient assignment care system, *International Journal of Nursing Studies*, 24(2), 145–153.

Barker, P. (1987) Evaluation in nursing; The nurse as behaviour therapist, in Milne, D. (ed.) *Evaluating Mental Health Practice: Methods and Applications*, Croom Helm, London.

Barker, P., Davison, M., Turner, J. and Park, B. (1997) Intensive care for people with serious mental illness, *Nursing Standard* 11(34), 40–2.

Butterworth, C. A. (1987) Psychiatric nursing: Fumbling in a vacuum or grasping at opportunity, *Mental Health Nursing: The Journal of the Psychiatric Nurses Association*, 6 October.

Carder, E. R. and Hall, C. V. (1981) The professional stress syndrome, *Psychosomatics*, 22(8), 672.

Firth, H., McIntee, J., McKeown, P. and Britton, P. (1987) Professional depression, 'burnout' and personality in longstay nursing, *International Journal of Nursing Studies*, 24(3), 227–37.

Goffman, E. (1968) *Asylum: Essays on the Social Situation of Mental Patients and Other Inmates*, Penguin, Harmondsworth, UK.

Hare, J., Pratt, C. C. and Andrew, D. (1988) Predictors of burnout in professional nurses working in hospitals and nursing homes, *International Journal of Nursing Studies*, 25(2), 105–15.

Jones, G. J., Janman, K., Payne, R. L. and Rick, J. T. (1987) Some determinants of stress in psychiatric nursing, *International Journal of Nursing Studies*, **24**(2), 129–44.

Keith-Lucas, A. (1972) *Giving and Taking Help*, University of North Carolina Press, Chapel Hill.

Masson, J. (1989) *Against Therapy*, Collins, London.

Parkes, C. M. (1972) *Bereavement: Studies of Grief in Adult Life*, Penguin, Harmondsworth, UK.

Peplau, H. (1986) Hildegard Peplau: Grande Dame of Psychiatric Nursing (interview), *Geriatric Nursing*, **7**(6), 328–30.

Pryser, P. (1984) Existential impact of professional exposure to life-threatening or terminal illness, *Bulletin of the Menninger Clinic*, **48**, 357–67.

Ritter, S. (1989) *Bethlem Royal and Maudsley Hospital Manual of Clinical Psychiatric Nursing Principles and Procedures*, Harper & Row, London.

Rowe, D. (1989) Foreword, in Masson, J. (1989) op. cit.

Schwartz, M. S. and Shockley, E. L. (1956) *The Nurse and the Mental Patient: A Study in Interpersonal Relations*, Russell Sage Foundation, New York.

Sullivan, H. S. (1947) *Conceptions of Modern Psychiatry*, William A. White, Psychiatric Foundation, Washington DC.

Travelbee, J. (1971) *Interpersonal Aspects of Nursing*, F. A. Davis, New York.

Vanderpool, J. P. (1984) Stressful patient relationships and the difficult patient, in Krueger, P. N. (ed.) *Rehabilitation Psychology*, Aspen, Rockville, Md.

Welch, D. (1983) *A Voice Through a Cloud*, King Penguin, Harmondsworth, UK.

Clinical supervision in sick children's nursing

6

Barbara Elliott and Judith Ellis

INTRODUCTION

The nursing of children has been considered as separate and different from nursing adults throughout the profession's history. The Nurses Registration Act (1919) set up five separate parts to the Register of nurses, one of these parts being that containing the names of nurses trained in the nursing of sick children (Ministry of Health, 1919). The need for specific educational preparation for nurses wishing to care for children has continued to be recognized. The establishment in 1986 of children's nursing as one of the four specialist branches in Project 2000 has been followed by the validation of an ever-increasing number of graduate and masters level paediatric programmes. Recent debate on the role of generic education programmes often centres upon meeting employment needs through provision of generic nurses who can provide a flexible workforce, with few arguments put forward to challenge the view that separate educational programmes better meet children's needs.

If the need for specific educational provision is accepted and the ethos of life-long learning endorsed, it is essential to consider what particular aspects may distinguish supervision of children's nurses from supervision of nurses in other specialities. This chapter will firstly consider supervision applied to the paediatric setting and then examine two of the major components which support the uniqueness of supervision in children's nursing: play and the acceptance of non-professionals (mainly parents) as true partners in care. With *Vision for the Future* (DoH, 1993) nurses in all specialities have been asked to consider partnership with non-professionals, but due to the developmental nature of paediatric care, a family focus and involvement remains a central tenet of paediatric care (RCN, 1994).

The chapter discusses supervision in children's nursing and therefore focuses on sick children nursed not only in paediatric wards and units, but also, due to the increasingly seamless nature of paediatric care, culminates with a short section on sick children receiving appropriate nursing support at home (DoH, 1996).

CLINICAL SUPERVISION

The value for practitioners of establishing a model of clinical supervision has received extensive support and is accepted as a target for the future (DoH, 1993). Practitioners are being encouraged to select a model of clinical supervision that provides personal and professional support and that ensures development of nursing that meets patient needs.

Over 30 years ago, Pettes (1967) described supervision as a process by which one practitioner was accountable to another practitioner to help him practise to the best of his ability. Developments in supervision increasingly attempt to recognize the individual accountability of all practitioners. Practitioners are being encouraged to adopt models of clinical supervision that allow professional exchange to enable the development of professional skills (Butterworth and Faugier, 1995) rather than hierarchical or, indeed, dictatorial enforcement. This exchange may, for example in child protection cases, occur not only between nurses but also between other members of the interagency/multi-disciplinary team.

An area of confusion that supports the misguided ethos that nurses must be supervised by senior nurses is that many practitioners still readily relate supervision to educational assessment (Neary, 1997). In such a situation, the role of the supervisor is said to be 'to respond to the perceived needs of the student or new recruit and to provide learning opportunities appropriate to those needs' (Jarvis, 1984). The best person to fulfil the role of supervisor in this context has long been debated and many would agree with Kenworthy and Nicklin (1989) that the only credible and professionally acceptable person to function in this capacity is the practising nurse – for children's nurse students, a children's nurse.

As the use of supervision is extended beyond achieving professional competencies for initial registration to take into account the provision of patient-focused care and the need for life-long learning, the issue of who should supervise is far more concerned with finding the right supervisor for a meaningful exchange about the area under consideration. For example, depending on the scenario, supervision may be best provided by a health visitor, social worker, psychologist, etc. – the list is extensive but all are professionals involved in clinical practice with the client group.

Selection of a model of supervision further highlights this issue. In some areas, if supervision is to be managerial, the supervisors may no longer be in practice and indeed supervision may again be viewed as a hierarchical or indeed judgmental encounter by an individual unable to exchange professional clinical expertise. This supports the selection and development of peer supervision where the onus remains upon practitioners sharing and supporting development with peers in some areas from different professional groups. For example, key workers in paediatric respite care and rehabilitation services may come from many different professional groups. Peer supervision not only requires individuals to accept being accountable for their own actions and professional development in safeguarding and promoting the interests of individual patients and clients (UKCC, 1992), but also their responsibilities in appropriately supporting their colleagues.

Many in nursing claim that supervision has always occurred, but the support of students, qualified new recruits, now formalized with preceptorship, and the hierarchical guidance that continues to be offered is now complemented by meaningful exchange between autonomous, accountable practitioners throughout professional practice. Through clinical supervision, supervisory commitment has become an integral part of life-long learning. It allows any practitioner involved in a therapeutic relationship with a patient or client to step back and evaluate the effectiveness of that relationship. Supervision may provide the objective validation of the helping relationship, which is of great importance to experienced practitioners as well as novices (Sundeen et al., 1985).

Children's nurses, like other nurses, have been slow to formalize the supervisory relationship for practitioners other than students. Indeed forms of supervision have at times been so subtle as to be undetectable. Supervision within the paediatric setting should be accepted, not only for its restorative value but also as it is essential for the maintenance and delivery of high standards of care.

Barber (1987) describes formal and informal supervision. The primary task of formal supervision is the supervision itself, but in informal supervision the primary task is the delivery of care. The suggestion is that informal supervision, when supervisor and supervisee work alongside each other, enables continuous and immediate exchange which is less threatening than formal supervision. Between peers this scenario is easily accepted as clinical supervision. However, if the colleague is the nurse in charge of the ward, responsible for allocating patient care to appropriate staff, this encounter rather than being viewed as informal supervision is in danger of appearing judgemental, an assessment of each staff member's level of ability and competence. It should be viewed by all as a valuable, informal, clinical supervision scenario with all acting as supportive colleagues.

In children's nursing this informal supervision is even more difficult to achieve because of the nature of care required. Nursing care of adult patients frequently requires two nurses: to bed bath, turn or lift a patient, for example. This gives the supervisor, be he or she a senior nurse or a peer, an ideal opportunity to work with the supervisee in a non-threatening way. Both the supervisor and supervisee can identify practical and interpersonal skills offering support and guidance, thus developing clinical skills and care and enhancing the exchange of ideas between professionals. Feedback may be immediate or delayed, but together they can identify areas to be developed.

Care of children frequently requires only one nurse and the supervisor and supervisee may feel awkward, having no other reason for being together than that they wish to undertake supervision. With experience, the supervisor may be able to ensure that her presence is not intrusive, but like the non-participant observer in research, her unease may at first compel her to take over care, or her very presence may make the situation unnatural and make the supervisee, patient, and indeed parents, feel ill at ease. The parent or child, as the receivers of care, may in fact provide the answer, being able to offer invaluable insight into a nurse's practice, if as partners they feel able to participate in reflection on particular care practices.

During preceptorship or a structured orientation period, direct and actual observation of practice is accepted if not expected and welcomed, with both preceptor and preceptee feeling at ease with informal supervision. However, on completion of preceptorship, the supervisor may find herself reliant upon the staff member directly seeking active supervision or on delayed supervision bringing issues to formally organized sessions. The emphasis in paediatrics must, therefore, be upon fostering, during preceptorship and orientation, a clear understanding of the usefulness of seeking out supervision, and in creating a supportive and non-judgmental atmosphere where all staff are mutually supportive. Staff at all levels of paediatric experience must not be reluctant to request informal supervision whether the supervisor is a peer or more senior member of staff, and must not see informal supervision as inferred criticism of her ability and interference with her nursing care.

An alternative to this one-to-one supervision is group supervision or indeed peer review. This may take place at hand-over reports, ward meetings, group sessions or multi-disciplinary case conferences and is often delayed supervision, reflecting back upon an event or practice that occurred earlier. Such meetings, as well as allowing discussion about specific care episodes, or supporting individual care practices, provide an excellent opportunity to focus upon general policies and standards. There is little evidence as yet, however, that such meetings formalize peer review or supervision, but an awareness of the potential of developing such meetings to fulfil a normative or indeed formative function, for example the development of protocols and policies, should be recognized.

It is vital that every opportunity to introduce supervision is grasped, particularly as limits on available time is often quoted by nurses as all that is preventing the existence of supervision. With minimal adaptation, what has previously been considered discussion may be formalized to achieve recognition as supervision. Indeed just because a meeting is not entitled supervision does not mean supervision cannot form an element of such a meeting.

Multi-disciplinary meetings, where the care of individual or groups of patients is discussed, may be another opportunity for formal supervision. Such meetings are usually held to discuss children with the same or similar diseases and are aimed at combining information from different sources and encouraging a united approach to care. This form of multi-disciplinary supervision is very valuable and provides a forum for discussion, reflection and objective evaluation for all levels of staff, and indeed it may be of value to consider parents in the multi-disciplinary discussion.

PLAY

One of the major differences between a children's and an adult ward is the noise and level of activity. Indeed, the uninitiated are often amazed at the apparent chaos and commotion of a children's ward. This state of affairs is usually the result of play in its many forms. This is the context within which the majority of paediatric nurses practise and the vital role and functions of play must be recognized in any discussion of paediatric care including supervision.

Psychologists have examined the functions of play in childhood and each has her or his own perspective on its importance. Whatever the perspective, there is an agreement that, as well as being pleasurable and intensely absorbing, play is essential for the development of the child's physical, psychological and social functioning and well-being.

Children in hospital must therefore be encouraged to play in order to continue their normal development, for as Wall states in Weller (1980), 'the child who cannot play is as severely threatened as the child who is deprived of nourishment'. In addition, for the child in hospital diversionary play may be the one normal element in an otherwise abnormal environment (Save the Children, 1989).

Play is also essential for the hospitalized child as a means of expressing her or his emotions and enabling him to make sense of what is happening to him. The effect of play on the psychological well-being of young children in hospital was studied by Noble (1967). She found that, in wards where there was no special provision for play, the children demonstrated most signs of disturbance. Play is one of the most powerful and effective means of stress reduction for children and is an important therapeutic tool for hospitalized children (Petrillo and Sanger, 1985; Sadler,

1990), a tool that needs to be fully utilized by all professionals involved in care.

For children's nurses play is also the means by which they can communicate with their young patients, gain their trust and encourage their co-operation (Weller, 1980; D'Antonio, 1984). Communication with children is essential in order to explain what is happening to them and what will happen in the future, in order to reduce their anxiety. Klinzing and Klinzing (1977) state that the primary reason for fear amongst hospitalized children is lack of understanding, but they warn that any means of providing information must take account of the child's intellectual ability.

A number of research studies cited by Hart et al. (1992) have lent support to the value of play for hospitalized children. The use of therapeutic play in providing children with information about their hospital stay, medical and surgical procedures and helping them deal with their emotions has been frequently documented (Knudsen, 1975; Azarnoff and Flegal, 1975; Rodin, 1983; D'Antonio, 1984; Chambers, 1993). The benefits of play for hospitalized children are not disputed. Indeed, play should not only be available, but all personnel involved in caring for sick children must use it to its full potential.

The DHSS (1976a) accepted the therapeutic advantage of encouraging play among children in hospital and suggested that play become part of nurses' work with children. Until this time the clinical model had dominated nurse training and the emphasis of nursing care was on the physical care of child patients, keeping the wards neat and tidy and minimising noise (Hawthorn, 1974). The ability to facilitate play and use it as a means of building a therapeutic relationship with child patients is now a recognised skill of the children's nurse. However, like talking to adult patients, play is often given low priority and is only to be indulged in after the 'work' is completed. Nurses may frequently be called away from playing in order to carry out clinical duties. Over the years, studies of children's nursing have shown that nurses spend very little time playing with their young patients and that they lack knowledge of children's play needs (Pill, 1970; Hawthorn, 1974; Hall, 1977; Rodin, 1983; Cross and Swift, 1990).

The eventual introduction of play workers to children's wards has improved the opportunities for children to play. There is, however, rarely a member of play staff available for the full 24 hours and nationally-accepted staffing recommendations of one play worker to ten children (Hogg, 1990) fails to take into account children in isolation or children requiring intensive play therapy. Save the Children (1989) recognized that the:

'special functions of play in the life of the child in hospital cannot be achieved unless an appropriately trained play specialist is present and unless the play specialist is working as an integral member of the paediatric team.' (Save the Children, 1989, p. 30)

The acceptance of play staff by nursing colleagues and the utilization of their special skills and knowledge has not been automatic. Hall found that nursing staff were reluctant to give the play leaders medical information and thus maintained a distinction between the care of sick children in the ward and the occupation of less ill children in the playroom (Hall, 1979). The nurses therefore failed to utilize the play leaders' skills. They unanimously agreed that play was a part of their, the nurses, duties, but observation suggested that when they were busy it was one of their lowest priorities and that, when they were less busy, they did not possess the knowledge or experience to be able to perform the role.

Nursing staff caring for children need to have the knowledge and skills to continue provision of play planned by, but in the absence of, qualified play staff. Play is an integral part of the education of children's nurses, but children's nurses need to accept the play staff's specialist expertise and knowledge, accepting them as professionals (Save the Children, 1989; Hogg, 1990) who provide an essential, complementary service and who can support them in life-long learning in this important area of care. Both groups would benefit from exchanges within a framework of clinical supervision, recognizing the two-way relationship of supervision. This would, in addition, assist play workers who are often the only play personnel involved in a particular care scenario where play may have been the main therapeutic intervention. For example, play therapy is increasingly being used with children who have behavioural and emotional problems, and this can involve the play worker in a very intense relationship with the child. Although such play staff will have received special training for this job, they nevertheless need supervision to evaluate their relationship and to discuss possible initiatives and progress. It is recommended that children's hospitals employ a senior play specialist to co-ordinate play staff (Hogg, 1990) and they could perhaps take on some of the supervisory role. However, it is unlikely that, if employed at all, such a person would be able to provide regular supervision for all play staff, a managerial model may also be inappropriate and, in practice, the relative isolation and lack of career structure within their own profession means that the play workers frequently rely on children's nurses to fulfil this role.

The vital role that play has in the care and treatment of children must be recognized, as once accepted as an important part of the children's nurse's role, peer supervision involving play and nursing staff can be seen as appropriate, with both parties contributing as an exchange between equals.

PARENTAL PARTICIPATION IN CARE

The greatest transformation in the care of sick children to which children's nurses have had to react and change their role has been the presence, and now participation, of parents in care (Coyne, 1995). In few areas of nursing are non-professionals so closely involved in care as in paediatrics. Darbyshire (1993), Palmer (1993) and Coyne (1995) have written comprehensive reviews of the literature on the history of parental involvement in the hospital care of children.

Parents are increasingly encouraged to continue the normal care that they would give to their child at home during his or her hospital admission. However, there is still no general consensus amongst children's nurses about the extent or form of parental participation (Callery and Smith, 1991) and there is evidence that nurses still have difficulty with parental participation (Darbyshire, 1994). This evidence alone raises a vital area for clinical supervision amongst all professionals caring for children and their families.

Normal childcare, often termed 'family care' (Casey, 1988; 1993), may be all that the parents are willing or able to do, and no pressure should be put upon them to do more. Reflection within supervision may help professionals recognize why unacceptable pressure is exerted. Many parents are increasingly learning to give nursing care, that is care relating to the health needs of the child, such as giving naso-gastric feeds, tracheotomy care, changing dressings, etc. Indeed, involvement of parents in nursing care is seen as a natural progression and of benefit to children, parents, medical and nursing staff (Webb *et al.*, 1985; Sainsbury *et al.*, 1986; Bishop, 1988; Goodwin, 1988; Taylor and O'Connor, 1989; Callery and Smith, 1991; Darbyshire, 1994). However, this assumption that parental participation in care is desirable reflects the changing expectations and attitudes amongst health-care professionals towards the role of parents in the care of the child. Supervision which involves parents may challenge even this assumption or expectation.

The relationship between the care that is given by the children's nurse and that which is given by the parents is often in a delicate balance. The nurse must carefully negotiate with parents the care that they wish to give and feel confident giving, the care which they require help with, the nursing care that they would like to learn to give and the care that they would never be happy giving under any circumstances. The nurse must be wary of leaving the parent to give family care without support when the child's condition means that their normal competence and confidence is impaired, for example leaving the parent to dress a child who has an intravenous infusion, or where they may feel unsure and insecure merely because of the strange environment, for example the hospital ward (Coyne, 1995). The process of nurses and parents negotiating roles is not without problems, and it cannot be assumed that all nurses are willing and able to negotiate (Callery and Smith, 1991). This needs the type of discussion supported by supervision.

Attempts are being made to formalize this relationship in terms of developing a model of nursing which incorporates parental and nursing interventions (Casey, 1988). The essential ingredients of this relationship must be communication and partnership, both areas for supervision.

This situation of non-professionals delivering care to the child, be it family care or nursing care, has implications for clinical supervision in children's nursing. Not only will issues around parental partnership be raised during formal supervision between professionals, but it may be postulated that if parents are true partners they may themselves play a key role both as supervisors and supervisees in informal and possibly formal supervision. Implications will be considered in two sections:

- parents as supervisors;
- supervising parents.

Parents as supervisors

In most situations the sick child's parents may be regarded as the experts in family care (Campbell and Summersgill, 1993). They know their child better than anyone else. They know his (or her) likes and dislikes, his normal routines and favourite games. A junior nurse may feel threatened by an experienced, confident mother, but who better to supervise her, and indeed all professional carers in learning new skills of family care, than that expert mother? Parents can usually see through a nurse's pretence at being experienced in childcare when she is not and would feel much more confident in trusting their child's care to a nurse whom they have already supervised giving that care. Even the experienced nurse will benefit from working with the child's parents as that experience may not be directly related to that individual child's and family's needs. It is unrealistic to expect parents to keep a constant vigil by their child's bedside, but occasionally parents dare not leave even for a cup of coffee because they fear that no one will know what to do if their child cries. This may not be viewed as an exchange between professionals, but in the care of that particular child the parents are certainly the experts.

The situation is often more apparent with children with physical and/or learning disabilities. The parents of these children are often already experts in aspects of nursing care and cope by having regular routines for such problems as elimination. Their child may have difficulties in communicating his needs and the parents have to become experts in interpreting facial expressions, movements or sounds. When such children are admitted to hospital, particularly if it is an unfamiliar ward, there may be role conflicts between their families and nurses. Ferraro and Longo (1985) suggest that these role conflicts are caused by the competency and confidence which families have developed through caring for their sick child and the usual model of care for acutely ill children encountered on the ward. It may be asserted that these very competent mothers prefer to continue giving all of their child's care and the nurse may take on a passive role. This may well be so, but it may also be that the parents do not trust the nurses to deliver care of an equal standard in their absence. If these parents were encouraged to spend a few hours exchanging knowledge and skills with a children's nurse caring for their child they might then feel confident enough to take a much needed break whilst their child is in hospital.

Parents who are taught to give technical nursing or medical care, such as intravenous drug administration, are taught the very high standards demanded by hospital protocols. They become technical experts; their technique having to be so continually perfect as to ensure that on discharge standards are not lowered. On subsequent hospital admissions the care may be taken over for a short period by medical or nursing staff, which may lead to problems. Doctors, in particular, may be unaware of the parent's knowledge and skills and may become indignant if their technique is criticized by the parents. Parents supervising care in this manner may be seen as threatening by staff, but in fact it can ensure scrupulous adherence to correct procedure and policy – true normative and indeed formative supervision (Proctor, 1992).

It is noteworthy that children receiving long-term treatment also become experts in their own care. They may not be able to undertake the care themselves but quietly supervise the hospital staff. A hesitant, unconfident or inexperienced practitioner is soon exposed by children who are not reticent in telling a doctor or nurse when they are not performing skills to the required standard!

Supervising parents

A number of children are admitted to hospital because the family care given by parents is not of a sufficiently high standard to prevent ill-health or because they require nursing or medical care to meet their health needs. Parents will then need careful assessment of their capabilities and learning needs. If parents are to contribute to the care of their sick child, the level of their contribution must be decided, as described earlier, and a programme of education and supervision devised. This may involve supervising family care, such as the sterilization of feeding equipment for a young baby, or nursing care, such as the management of a raised temperature. Children's nurses need to use all their counselling and supervisory skills to enable parents to develop their full potential.

In some 'care by parents schemes', such as described by Cleary (1992), the nurse's main function is to teach, support and council parents who deliver and record all their child's care. Such schemes have been very successful in terms of reducing the time children are alone and awake or crying and ensuring that the majority of their contacts are with a family member, usually their mother (Cleary, 1992). Medical and nursing staff have also found such schemes satisfactory, but to date they have been slow to develop in the UK.

The role of parents in the care of sick children will continue to develop (Coyne, 1995). Children's nurses must therefore continue to reassess their role with parents and be prepared to accept supervision from parents and in return give such supervision to them as the changing situation demands. Exchange between practitioners is occurring, even if parents are only the practitioners with their own child.

CARE OF THE SICK CHILD IN THE COMMUNITY

Throughout the UK, services are being developed to support parents in caring for their sick child at home (RCN, 1993a). The need for such services was highlighted in the Platt Report (Ministry of Health, 1959) with a drive for many years to only admit children to hospital if the care they require cannot be as well provided at home (DHSS, 1976b; DoH, 1991). This change in service provision is not only seen as benefiting the child and family by maintaining normal social functioning and relationships, but also as a more cost-effective option (DoH, 1996). There is no uniformity in the structure and organization of these services, but all are seeking to employ children's qualified nurses (RCN, 1993b).

For some, namely those on Part 15 of the UKCC register, their training was designed to equip them to function within the community, but for many their training was focused upon care of a sick child in a hospital setting. Educational programmes are being developed to assist the staff in this transition, but for many services, who employ minimal numbers of children's qualified staff, it is difficult if not impossible to release staff to complete these programmes. Supervision for these nurses is of vital importance but may be complex in nature as, especially until peer supervision is readily available and the services are well-established, many could be seen as having a vital role to play in such supervision, for example, all members of the primary and acute hospital care teams, occasionally specialist paediatric centres, education services, social services and indeed parents and the children. Such multi-disciplinary/ multi-agency supervision would certainly support development of an interagency team, but may also give rise to professional rivalry and protectionism.

CONCLUSION

Sick children have their own unique problems and needs, and their nursing care requires skills quite different from those required for nursing adults. In this chapter three areas in children's nursing have been discussed which require specialist skills and education for practising nurses and raise issues regarding clinical supervision for those nurses. An attempt has been made to address some of those issues and suggestions made for the future of clinical supervision in children's nursing. There are, of course, many other aspects to the specialist area of paediatric nursing and the future development of degree and masters level programmes, children's community nursing services and true interdisciplinary patient-focused care will provide further areas for consideration.

Sick children's nursing continues to develop. Children will continue to have special needs and clinical supervision will support all professionals, but particularly children's nurses, in meeting these needs in whatever context care is delivered.

REFERENCES

Azarnoff, P. and Flegal, S. (1975) *A Paediatric Play Programme*, Charles C. Thomas, Illinois.

Barber, P. (1987) Skills in supervision, *Nursing Times*, 14 Jan., 56–7.

Bishop, J. (1988) Sharing the caring, *Nursing Times*, **84**(30), 60–1.

Butterworth, T. and Faugier, J. (1995) *Clinical Supervision in Nursing, Midwifery and Health Visiting. A Briefing Paper*, University of Manchester, Manchester.

Callery, P. and Smith, L. (1991) A study of role negotiation between nurses and the parents of hospitalised children, *Journal of Advanced Nursing*, **16**, 772–81.

Campbell, S. and Summersgill, P. (1993) Putting the family first, *Child Health*, **1**(2), 59–63.

Casey, A. (1988) A partnership with child and family, *Senior Nurse*, **8**(4), 8–9.

Casey, A. (1993) Developing a model for paediatric nursing practice, pp. 183–93, in Glasper, A. and Tucker, A. (eds) *Advances in Child Health Nursing*, Scutari, London.

Chambers, M. A. (1993) Play as therapy for the hospitalised child, *Journal of Clinical Nursing*, **2**, 349–54.

Cleary, J. (1992) *Caring for Children in Hospital: Parents and Nurses in Partnership*, Scutari, London.

Coyne, I. T. (1995) Parental participation in care: A critical review of the literature, *Journal of Advanced Nursing*, **21**, 716–22.

Cross, C. A. and Swift, P. G. F. (1990) Observation and measurements of play activities on a paediatric ward, *Maternal and Child Health*, Dec., 354–61.

D'Antonio, I. J. (1984) Therapeutic use of play in hospitals, *Nursing Clinics of North America*, **19**(2), 351–9.

Darbyshire, P. (1993) Parents, nurses and paediatric nursing: A critical review, *Journal of Advanced Nursing*, **18** 1670–80.

Darbyshire, P. (1994) *Living with Sick Children in Hospital: The Experiences of Parents and Nurses*, Chapman & Hall, London.

DHSS (1976a) *The Report of the Expert Group on Play on Hospital*, HMSO, London.

DHSS (1976b) *Fit for the Future: Report of the Court Committee on Child Health Services*, HMSO, London.

DoH (1991) *Welfare of Children and Young People in Hospital*, HMSO, London.

DoH (1993) *A Vision for the Future: The Nursing, Midwifery and Health Visiting Contribution to Health and Health Care*, HMSO, London.

DoH (1996) *Child Health in the Community*, HMSO, London.

Ferraro, A. R. and Longo, D. C. (1985) Nursing care of the family with a chronically ill, hospitalised child. An alternative approach, *Image*, **17**(2), 77–81.

Goodwin, P. (1988) 'I know you're busy but . . .', *Nursing Times*, **84**(30), 62.

Hall, D. J. (1977) *Social Relations and Innovation Changing the State of Play in Hospitals*, Routledge & Kegan Paul, London.

Hall, D. J. (1978) Bedside blues: The impact of social research on the hospital treatment of sick children, *Journal of Advanced Nursing*, **3**(1), 25–37.

Hart, R., Mather, P. L., Slack, J. F. and Powell, M. A. (1992) *Therapeutic Play Activities for Hospitalised Children*, Mosby Year Book Inc., St Louis.

Hawthorn, P. (1974) *Nurse – I Want My Mummy*. RCN, London.

Hogg, C. (1990) *Quality Management for Children: Play in Hospital*, Play in Hospital Liaison Committee, London.

Jarvis, P. (1984) The educational role of the supervisor in the tutorial relationship. *Nurse Education Today*, **3**(6), 126–9.

Kenworthy, N. and Nicklin, P. (1989) *Teaching and Assessing in Nursing and Practice: An Experiential Approach*, Scutari Press, London.

Klinzing, D. R. and Klinzing, R. G. (1977) *The Hospitalised Child: Communication Techniques for Health Personnel*, Prentice-Hall, New Jersey.

Knudsen, K. (1975) Play therapy: Preparing the young child for surgery, *Nursing Clinics of North America*, **10**(1), 679–86.

Ministry of Health for England and Wales (1919) *Nurses Registration Act*, HMSO, London.

Ministry of Health (1959) *The Welfare of Children in Hospital (the Platt Report)*, HMSO, London.

Neary, M. (1997) Defining the role of assessors, mentors and supervisors, *Nursing Standard*, **11**(42), 34–7.

Noble, E. (1967) *Play and the Sick Child*, Faber, London.

Palmer, S. J. (1993) Care of sick children by parents: A meaningful role, *Journal of Advanced Nursing*, **18**, 185–91.

Pettes, D. E. (1967) *Supervision in Social Work: A Method of Student Training and Staff Development*, National Institute for Social Work Training, Series No. 10, Allen & Unwin, London.

Petrillo, M. and Sanger, S. (1985) *Emotional Care of Hospitalised Children*, 3rd edition, Lippincott, Philadelphia.

Proctor, B. (1992) On being a trainer and supervision for counselling in action, in

Hawkins, P. and Shoet, R. (eds) *Supervision in the Helping Professions*, Open University Press, Milton Keynes, UK.

Pill, R. (1970) The sociological aspects of the case study sample, in Stacey, M. (ed.) *Hospitals, Children and Their Families*, Routledge & Kegan Paul, London.

Rodin, J. (1983) *Will This Hurt? Preparing Children for Hospital and Medical Procedures*, RCN, London.

RCN (1993a) *Directory of Paediatric Community Nursing Services*, 10th edition, RCN, London.

RCN (1993b) *Buying Paediatric Community Nursing: A Guide for Purchasers and Commissioners of Health Care* RCN, London.

RCN (1994) *The Care of Sick Children: A Review of the Guidelines in the Wake of the Allitt Inquiry*, RCN, London.

Sadler, C. (1990) Child's play, *Nursing Times*, **86**(11), 16–17.

Sainsbury, C. P. Q., Gray, O. P., Cleary, J. *et al.* (1986) Care by parents of their children in hospital, *Archives of Disease in Childhood*, **61**, 612–15.

Save the Children (1989) *Hospital: A Deprived Environment for Children. The Case for Hospital Play Schemes*, Save the Children, London.

Sundeen, S. J., Stuart, G. W., Rankin, E. and Cohen, S. (1985) *Nurse Client Interaction*, Mosby, St Louis.

Taylor, M. R. H. and O'Connor, P. (1989) Resident parents and shorter hospital stay, *Archives of Disease in Childhood*, **64**(2), 274–6.

UKCC (1992) *Code of Professional Conduct for Nurses, Midwives and Health Visitors* 3rd edition, UKCC, London.

Webb, N., Hull, D. and Madeley, R. (1985) Care by parents in hospital, *British Medical Journal*, **291**, 176–7.

Weller, B. F. (1980) *Helping Sick Children Play*, Baillière Tindall, London.

Developing supervision in adult/general nursing

7

Carol Marrow and Talib Yaseen

'Pooh began to feel a little more comfortable, because when you are a Bear of Very Little Brain, and you Think of Things, you find sometimes that a Thing which seemed very Thingish inside you is quite different when it gets out into the open and has other people looking at it.'

(Milne, 1928)

INTRODUCTION

The quotation above from a well-known children's book, does not in any way infer that nurses have *little brains*. However, it does suggest that some nurses display little confidence in their abilities, and are therefore reluctant to share their feelings and ideas with others. Perhaps this is because of their perceived lack of knowledge on professional issues, which can all too often result in stultified practice. Sharing ideas and issues is a means of helping to relieve emotional tension, aid clarification of thoughts and promote experimentation on, and sometimes changes in, practice. Nurses are developing their professional skills and knowledge. They are also beginning to engage in professional dialogue, especially through the promotion of ideas in action, such as reflective practice and clinical supervision. However, these concepts are taking time to assimilate into the clinical nursing culture. This is considered to be partly related to the hierarchical system of nursing management which prevailed until recent times.

This chapter intends to review briefly the past and current supervisory practice in adult general nursing. It will then present an overview of an ongoing action research study on clinical supervision and reflective practice in various adult nursing clinical settings and further illustrate the early findings of this empirical work.

NURSING THE ADULT PATIENT

'Adult nursing' is an umbrella term that encompasses a complex range of specialist nursing skills, including the care of medical patients, surgical patients, patients in high-dependency units, and the care of older people to name a few. The clinical contexts within adult general nursing are very complex, both organizationally and conceptually. Although specialist fields are now more apparent within the nursing profession, there is, however, some confusion regarding these roles and to aid clarity this chapter aims to focus on all aspects of adult nursing environments. Many nurses working in these clinical settings have been socialized into beauracratic and hierarchical systems of management, resulting in an overemphasis on nursing tasks and rituals, (Walsh and Ford, 1989). Within these hierarchical structures, tasks were delegated to the able individual who would carry them out according to their level of expertise and responsibility. Monitoring of junior staffs' competencies was evident through many supervisory roles. There existed different levels of nursing staff, including auxiliary nurses. These were and are seen as the lowest in the ranks and carry out fundamental aspects of care intervention under the supervision of a qualified nurse. Above the auxiliary nurses were the student nurses, whom Melia described as often being used interchangeably with the auxiliary nurse (Melia 1987). Then followed the qualified nurses, including the practical trained enrolled nurse and the more theoretically trained registered nurse. The registered nurses had a hierarchy of their own from junior staff nurse, senior staff nurse, ward charge nurse or sister to the nurse line managers.

Many changes within nursing practice have instigated a shift from task-orientated care. Concepts such as individualized care, critical pathways, primary nursing and, not least, the 'named nurse' have all had an impact on the management of patient care.

One implication of this move away from delegated tasks is the reliance on the skills, knowledge and judgement of the nurse to deliver the individualized care that a given patient requires. Nurses do exercise a high level of individual judgement about the needs of individual patients. However, from the experience gained from introducing the 'named nurse' concept, it is not without its problems. The culture of nursing appears to remain one where nurses are not confident to debate, nor justify, the quality of nursing delivered.

The role of the ward sister has also changed significantly over the last few years. Many senior staff appear confused about their overall responsibility for the care delivered to the patients, and the level of accountability and autonomy available to an individual nurse. A framework of supervision could be of value in clarifying such matters.

SUPERVISION TO DATE IN ADULT NURSING PRACTICE: THE HISTORICAL PERSPECTIVE

Nursing appears to have some history of clinical supervisory practice, although not specifically under the guise of mentorship, preceptorship or clinical supervision. One example of this was student nurses who, throughout their training, were often overseen whilst carrying out patient care. Midwifery has used superintendent midwives for supervision for over nine decades and community nursing has included fieldwork supervision. Moreover, as far back as Florence Nightingale in the 1800s, the learners' first-year practical nursing took place in hospital under supervision (Palmer, 1983). Recent times have seen the inception of the clinical teachers' role. Even more recently, we have witnessed the introduction of the role of the clinical mentor for students, the preceptor role for newly qualified nurses and clinical supervision for all qualified nurses.

WHY SUPERVISION FOR ADULT NURSING?

For decades other professions, such as social work, counselling, teaching and psychiatry, have used formal systems of supervision to support both their novice practitioners and even their experienced practitioners (Kurpious *et al.*, 1977). Nursing in adult care has been reticent to take on formal supervisory roles, even though high levels of stress are evident within the profession. This has resulted in high sickness as well as high attrition rates (Kramer, 1974). However, the Chief Nursing Officer at the Department of Health (DoH) is now urging the profession both to debate the notion of clinical supervision and to develop frameworks for practice. Butterworth (Butterworth and Faugier, 1992), expresses the view that nurses should have supervision for life from mentorship to preceptorship, and then clinical supervision, to help promote better standards of care through critical enquiry.

Mentorship

Mentorship within UK adult nursing has mainly concentrated on student nurses. In 1987, 1988 and 1989 the English National Board (ENB) directed training institutions to ensure that all clinical environments where students trained had implemented a system of mentorship. The ENB did not appear to be specific regarding the content and duration of the training and development of these mentors. Thus, health authorities and schools of nursing differed in their delivery of these courses, resulting in a variety of standards. That said, although beset with problems, this system has on occasions been successful, with student nurses having some form of support and guidance whilst on their clinical placements. The role has also been of value to qualified nurses by helping promote their professional development. However, as already suggested, the quality of the mentor relationship has varied within clinical environments, from a high level of effective support to very little interaction between the mentor and the student (Jacka and Lewin, 1987; ENB, 1993; Marrow, 1995; Cahill, 1996). Examples from a recent research study are given here:

Observation notes:

'The student is working on an early shift on this ward. She has been working alone most of the morning. Difficult to observe supervision as it does not appear to be occurring. She has worked a little with a third year student nurse, but sister seems to be around and overseeing. This student, however, is in the very early stages of her training and should not be left for the length of time observed (3 hours).' (Marrow, 1995, p. 100)

A student's comment from the interview notes:

'Supervision could be improved if the staff had more time to do it, things are done at a fast pace and, therefore, you are not shown step by step, it's done very quickly and sometimes you can't really see what they are doing.' (Marrow, 1995, p. 100)

Other literature further highlights these issues and many others associated with the role (Darling, 1984; Burnard, 1988; Laurent, 1988; Donovan, 1990). More recent studies suggest that the aim of mentorship relationships is changing, with support as the most fundamental aspect of the role (Earnshaw, 1995). Nevertheless, students participating in a recent study suggest that in the future a more challenging approach to the supervisory process will emerge (Cameron-Jones and O'Hara, 1996), hence having implications on the way mentors and supervisors in the future are trained and developed.

Preceptorship

The preceptor roles for newly qualified nurses and nurses returning to practice have been adopted in the UK through the recommendations of the PREP report (UKCC, 1990) and local policies. These recommendations would seem to be problematic as the PREP requirements are not a statutory obligation, but evidence of good practice. Many health-care trusts and hospitals do not always appear committed to the concept of preceptorship, as evidenced by the lack of clear protocols for preceptorship practice. Valid reasons for this lack of commitment may exist, not least over-stretched budgets and low morale in the clinical areas.

The literature, to date, on preceptorship in the UK shows a lack of rigorous evaluation of the process and outcomes of the notion in action. That said, some evaluations of preceptor programmes have taken place (Allanach and Mowinski Jennings, 1990) and they have helped to raise our understanding of the role. This lack of empirical evidence, however, only serves to highlight the importance of implementing strategies that will rigorously evaluate preceptorship policies in practice. Although some hospitals and trusts are utilizing the concept in action, the style and approach vary widely. Some trusts offer, for the newly qualified practitioner, a type of induction programme. Others use the idea synonymously with assessment, where the preceptee is judged summatively on knowledge, attitude and skills. The reasons for these inconsistencies may be attributed to the vagueness of the UKCC's document.

In the United States preceptorship has been available for both pre-registration nurses and post-registration nurses for decades (Shamian and Lemieux, 1984; Myrick and Awrey, 1988; Scheetz, 1989; Ouellet, 1993). Many of the findings suggest that the effects of preceptorship on the individual practitioner are on the whole positive for a variety of reasons.

Although these studies are helpful, many of them have utilized a quasi-experimental research design. This approach limits the depth and breadth of the information provided. A fuller picture might have been revealed utilizing a more qualitative approach.

Clinical supervision

Various reports that advocate clinical supervision as a means to promoting effective nursing practice have been produced. These include *A Strategy for Nursing* (DoH, 1989) and *A Vision for the Future* (DoH, 1993). Others that also promote the concept are *Clinical Supervision: A Report of the Trust Nurse Executives Workshops* (Bishop, 1994) and *Clinical Supervision in Practice* (Kohner, 1994). Many of these reports are promoting the concept of clinical supervision for all practitioners. The *Vision for the Future* document directs the profession, through target 10, to explore, define and develop a clinical supervision strategy for practice. On evaluation of the results of this directive, outlined in the document *Testing the Vision* (DoH, 1994), there is evidence that many health authorities are in the process of exploring and discussing the idea of clinical supervision. Furthermore, in some instances, many are now testing the idea in practice. The clinical supervision workshops requested by the Trust Nurse Executives have been a positive step in the right direction, highlighting the interest and commitment to try to implement clinical supervision. The King's Fund document (Kohner, 1994) also reflects positive moves in the development of clinical supervision, albeit in ideal situations.

Other more recent literature on clinical supervision suggests that many models of clinical supervision are now being utilized in practice (Friedman and Marr, 1995; Ritter *et al.*, 1996). However, there is little empirical evidence yet available to evaluate their success concerning nurses' development and the standard of care that patients and clients receive. Thus, to convince managers and policy-makers of the value of supervision, substantial research in this area needs to be implemented and rigorously evaluated.

SUPERVISION IN AN ADULT NURSING SETTING: A SUMMARY OF A REGIONAL PILOT PROJECT

The clinical supervision project discussed here is part of a North West Regional pilot study. To promote a more rigorous evaluation of the pilot study, an action research approach was chosen and the action research will continue to investigate clinical supervision after the pilot has concluded and been evaluated. At the outset, the research involved ten case studies and included ten qualified nurses as supervisors and 20 qualified nurses as supervisees. These numbers later reduced to six case studies, incorporating six supervisors and 14 supervisees; the reasons for the decrease in numbers are commented upon later. The work has been ongoing for approximately 18 months. Data is obtained from focused group discussions and a repertory grid based on Kelly's Personal Construct Theory (Kelly, 1963).

The pilot study commenced with a request for volunteers to be supervisors. Preparatory workshops were organized for the volunteers to attend. These consisted of a two-day workshop and follow-up day to explore the notion of clinical supervision and reflective practice. A protocol for supervision in practice and user-friendly reflective diaries were also formalized. It is important to stress that ownership of the clinical supervision protocol came from the practitioners involved. This is a relevant issue, as practitioners need to feel that they have participated in policy decisions and that they fully support and understand the initiatives. The research protocol that evolved from the workshops included important elements essential for supervision to be successful. These incorporated an agreed definition of the term 'clinical supervision', aims of the project, the research questions and the prerequisite qualifications and experience. Other important aspects included ground rules for the supervisory sessions, the style and approach, and the means of evaluation.

The supervisees' workshops

Supervisees chosen by the supervisor attended half-day workshops. These were organized for the supervisees to explore and discuss the concepts of clinical supervision, reflective practice and the use of the reflective diary.

Agreed definition of clinical supervision

In the workshops, a consensus was reached that the ultimate aim of clinical supervision was the improvement of patient care. The potential supervisors worked in groups and each group formulated a definition of clinical supervision. The interpretations were later combined to form one ultimate meaning of the concept:

> ' "Clinical supervision aims to support, motivate and encourage personal and professional growth through the sharing of knowledge and experience". It consists of regular, structured meetings between practising professionals, based on mutual trust and respect in a caring and positive environment.' (Furness General Hospital, 1995)

The aim of the research

The aim of the research was identified and agreed by the group:

> ' "To provide a supportive and sharing relationship that empowers the individuals involved to reflect on their own competencies". This should enable the practitioners to develop both personally and professionally which would help to enhance standards of care and effectiveness of care management.' (Furness General Hospital, 1995)

The research question

The research question to be answered was:

> Is there evidence of an increase in the practitioner's knowledge and understanding of practice and supervision issues through the process of clinical supervision? If there is an indication of the above (question one) how is this demonstrated? For example: an improvement in problem-solving skills; an increase in both confidence and competence; evidence of an advance in theoretical knowledge and its application to practice; promotion of research awareness and utilization of research findings in practice.

This research question was originally identified by the research participants at the preparatory workshops and is therefore grounded in clinical practice. However, other personal constructs identified through exploratory interviews after completion of the workshops have been added to the list. These formed, along with the elements (learning contexts), the framework for one of the data collecting methods that is discussed later.

The prerequisite qualifications and experience of both the supervisor and supervisee

These requirements are both stated in the research protocol and were thus acted upon; the demands being that the qualified nurse had a minimum of 12 months experience and was both willing and motivated to take on the role of the clinical supervisor and complete a diary. They should also have attended a workshop on clinical supervision and have knowledge of Herons work (Heron, 1990).

The supervisee was also to be both willing and motivated to complete a reflective diary and discuss issues from that diary (as they choose). They should also have attended workshops that helped them to explore supervision issues and the utilization of the diary.

A catalogue of skills and attributes required by both the supervisor and supervisee were also included in the protocol. This list was quite extensive, but included counselling skills, managerial skills, research awareness, the ability to give and receive constructive criticism, problem-solving skills, willingness to accept change and keenness to develop.

Ground rules for action

To establish the relationship between supervisor and supervisee it was important that both parties fully understood the terms of the relationship. Butterworth suggests that:

> 'In a profession which embraces mentorship and supervision it is permissible to identify a number of ground rules.'
> (Butterworth, in Butterworth and Faugier, 1992, p. 12)

The important ground rules include confidentiality, timing and length of the sessions, the context and the process of clinical supervision. Other pertinent issues include notetaking and accessibility to information, respect for the person, the number of practitioners to be supervised and who will support the supervisors.

Style and approach

The style decided upon for this particular hospital trust was one-to-one supervision. However, if individuals felt strongly about another particular style of supervision, for example peer group supervision, then this choice was respected and supported.

The approach or model of supervision was based on the reflective cycle (Boud et al., 1985; Gibbs, 1988) and Heron's counselling intervention style (Heron, 1990). These are the frameworks for the reflective diaries and are discussed more fully later.

Evaluating the research pilot

To encourage a rigorous approach to the evaluation of both the process and outcomes of the clinical supervision project, a scientific approach to the data collection and analysis was decided upon.

Research methodology

Semi-structured interviews and questionnaires were originally the data collecting methods chosen, but were later rejected as they were not considered the best approach to meet the research aims. After careful consideration, structured interviews, utilizing a repertory grid technique and focused discussion groups, were the methods chosen.

Prior to the workshops, individuals were interviewed to ascertain their knowledge on clinical supervision and reflective practice. This helped to form a baseline for evaluation of the supervisors' perceived understanding of supervision prior to the workshops and the onset of the research in practice. After completion of the workshops, the research participants were encouraged to start their supervision sessions as soon as it was feasible.

Many of the participants began their supervisory interviews soon after the workshops had completed. The focused groups were started immediately and, after a two-month period, the individual interviews commenced.

Repertory grid technique

The grid is way of obtaining an individual's perceptions of other people, themselves and how they behave in different contexts.

This grid technique, based on Kelly's Personal Construct Theory (Kelly, 1967) has been utilized quite extensively in the psychology, education and management fields (Bannister and Fransella, 1977 and 1986; Stewart and Stewart, 1981; Beail, 1985). The idea is relatively new to the nursing profession, but does appear to have been a research tool of choice in some areas of nursing (Pollock, 1986; Morrison, 1989; Rawlinson, 1995).

The technique helps to reduce interviewer bias and considers the other research variables in the setting (Stewart & Stewart, 1981) and helps the research participants to interpret their world in a more scientific manner.

Ten learning contexts which included guided reflection, were identified and utilized in the grid (the term 'guided reflection' was the preferred choice of the research participants). Included also were ten personal constructs that had to be rated on each learning context on a scale of 1 to 5 (5 being the most positive). The ten clinical learning environments and the ten constructs were taken from interview transcripts. These interviews took place with a sample group of supervisors and supervisees to help

Element: Guided reflection

constructs

Not supported	1....................................5	Supported
Unmotivated	1....................................5	Motivated
Not empowered	1....................................5	Empowered
Not reflective	1....................................5	Reflective
Not knowledgeable	1....................................5	Knowledgeable
Not questioning	1....................................5	Questioning
Incompetent	1....................................5	Competent
Uncommunicative	1....................................5	Communicative
Not innovative	1....................................5	Innovative
Stressed	1....................................5	Not stressed

Figure 7.1 Rated element 'Guided reflection'

develop a repertory grid that was personal to the research participants. The learning environments are the important elements that the constructs are graded against. For example, the ten elements on the grid are identified as nursing handovers, team nursing, critical incidents, guided reflection, informal conversation, teaching others, patient interactions, the named nurse, courses and working on my own. The research participants have to rate how they feel they have developed through each of the elements. These personal ideas or mental framings are called 'constructs' and include motivated, supported, empowered, reflective, knowledgeable, questioning, competent, communicative, innovative and not stressed. To illustrate this the element 'guided reflection' is shown in Figure 7.1.

Focused group discussions

The focused group discussions were originally a means of support and supervision for the research participants. However, these groups developed far more than expected and became a valuable means of collecting data that could help evaluate the research project. The groups were tape-recorded to capture the intensity of the participant's feelings and to ensure that important information was not missed. To date, six focused discussion groups have taken place, three for the supervisors and three for the supervisees.

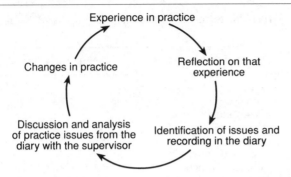

Figure 7.2 Cycle of reflection and supervision

Reflective diaries

The research diary format was written by the research facilitator. On the third day of the workshops, they were given to the study participants to allow critical evaluation of the content to take place, which resulted in some modification. The framework for the diaries was different for the supervisors and supervisees. The supervisor's diary aimed at analysing supervisory skills using Heron's model of intervention analysis (Heron, 1990). The six main interaction styles that Heron promotes are: prescriptive, informative, confronting, cathartic, catalytic and supportive. The research participants were encouraged to use other words that reflected similar meanings if they felt uncomfortable with the terminology.

The supervisees' framework was based on a reflective practice model extrapolated from various theoretical stances (Schon, 1983; Palmer *et al.*, 1994; Johns, 1994; Boud *et al.*, 1985). See Figure 7.2.

It must be emphasized that the diaries were used to help the participants focus on practice and supervision issues and were not utilized as data for the research findings. It is important to have a clear structure to work from at the outset of any study or project, otherwise those involved will flounder. Indeed, even with a firm framework the participants in this study did experience difficulties.

Evaluation of the process and outcome of supervision

Self- and peer evaluation with reflective diaries was encouraged throughout. Qualitative information was and still is being identified through the focused group discussions and the repertory grids. Quantitative data was and is being collected and analysed also through the repertory grids. To date, 12 supervisees have been interviewed using the repertory grid. The findings from these 12 indicate that the guided reflection element scores the most positive, compared to the other nine elements in seven out of the

Table 7.1 Construct 'Stressed' as rated in the different learning situations (elements)

	Stressed (1)	Not stressed (5)
Elements		
Handover		43
Team nursing		41
Critical incidents		31
Guided reflection		**54**
Informal conversation		46
Teaching others		46
Patient interaction		48
Named nurse		44
Courses		41
Working on my own		44

10 constructs. The seven constructs rating most positive are: motivated, supported, empowered, reflective, questioning, communicative and not stressed, with not stressed being the most positive score for guided reflection compared to the other nine clinical learning contexts, as highlighted in Table 7.1.

Caution is emphasized, as these are early findings from a proportion of the sample group. The research participants will all be interviewed on three further occasions and the final data will be analysed through both statistical analysis and qualitative content analysis.

Qualitative information extracted from the early focused discussion groups and exploratory interviews indicates that both the supervisors and supervisees have found clinical supervision beneficial as it enables the individuals participating to become more aware of their own feelings and practices. For example, one supervisor stated: 'it makes you more aware of yourself, it makes you a better practitioner. It makes you more reflective.'

Another supervisor:

'It can give you professional awareness in its broader sense. Within that, it will help you gain a different variety of skills, knowledge and different ways of thinking. In a particular sense it can give people support, real support in times of great difficulty. It could be instantaneous support, there and then or longer term. It will help you tease out the issues at that time.'

A supervisee:

'It always made me think. I knew I would be having a supervision session, so it made me reflect on issues in preparation. It has helped me maintain motivation rather than it wane off. The supervision kept that going.'

Although many of the findings, including the personal narratives from this study, are positive about clinical supervision, it is not without problems.

Practical difficulties with the implementation of clinical supervision

Many of the difficulties experienced by everyone engaged in the study need to be explored, as they have implications for the future implementation of clinical supervision in adult nursing.

Commitment to the study

Supervisors need to be committed to the concept of clinical supervision as it requires some generosity of themselves and this includes time and energy. For example one supervisor in the study stated: 'The interviews proved to be more successful when they were conducted in my "off duty" time and the supervisee was on duty.'

Some of the supervisors in this study have not always attended the focused groups and no reasons have been given for this. This may have caused problems for their supervisees who may have not received consistent supervision. There is at the present time total commitment from six of the original ten supervisors. Reasons for the reduction in actual supervision need to be explored further and evaluated, as this may have implications for future clinical supervision protocols. Indeed, Hart, Bond and Meyer suggest that often in action research projects, particularly in nursing fields, the involvement of participants in the research changes, can cause problems with commitment and continuity for the duration of the study (Meyer, 1993; Hart and Bond, 1995).

Quality of the supervision

The quality of supervision can vary and this can be due to the skills and commitment of the supervisor. Clinical experience is important, as is supervisory style. Using a format to help analyse interactional skills was beneficial in this study, as supervision is ultimately about identifying key issues through skilled communication techniques. Supervision is a difficult process to manage and therefore these important elements should not be under-estimated. At the outset, in-depth training and education of the supervisors should be implemented. This should be supported further with ongoing guidance and recognition.

Style of supervision

As already stated at the outset of this study, supervisors chose one-to-one supervision as the most appropriate style to implement. This has appeared to be difficult to implement on a large scale. The feasibility of every practising nurse having one-to-one supervision could be problematic without extra resources. Perhaps a combination of one-to-one (where individuals feel they need that for a given period of time) and peer group supervision could be advantageous. However, as supervision develops, individual practitioners should find different ways of being supervised to enhance their development. One such way could be self-supervision or self-appraisal as is implied in Scope of Professional Practice, paragraph 9.3 (UKCC, 1992):

> 'nurses must honestly acknowledge any limits of personal knowledge and skill and take steps to remedy any relevant deficits in order effectively and appropriately to meet the needs of patients and clients.'

Using the diaries

Many of the supervisees in this study found using the diaries difficult. They felt that they could articulate their feelings orally, but did not know where to begin when it came to recording the issues in writing. In fact, six months into the study, as some of the supervisees were still experiencing difficulties with using the diary, a one-day workshop was organized to help them explore the concept of reflective practice further and facilitate the appropriate recording of practice issues in a safe environment.

Reflecting on practice

Reflecting on practice is a valuable means of appraising care interventions and promoting problem-solving skills. However, reflection is a powerful tool and should not be underestimated in terms of personal and professional trauma. Highlighting difficulties and tensions on care issues can cause individuals much psychological distress. If we, as professionals, are requesting that nurses reflect on their care in a formal and structured way, then quality support should be made available to the practitioner to help deal with the issues. This will aid the practitioner in exploring these concerns in a safe and caring environment.

Taking responsibility

Initially, responsibility of organizing and leading the sessions was generally taken on board by the supervisor. However, it was understood that the supervisory relationship was a two-way interaction and no one person was in charge. It was therefore hoped that the supervisees would start to take the initiative and request supervision sessions, rather than this responsibility being the supervisors'. This has happened in some cases, but not in all. It does emphasize the importance of supervision being an obligation for both parties and that there is equal responsibility regarding the relationship.

Support for the supervisors and supervisees

Supporting individuals is essential throughout any process of change, and should be at its maximum in the early stages of any new implementation. Support was evident in this study, but some of the supervisors, for whatever reason, did not always request it. This was indicated by the lack of attendance at some of the supervisors' focused group meetings. Perhaps reasons for this could have been the presence of the nursing director, and the participants' perceived hierarchical group structure. Moreover, lack of time and staff may have also contributed to their lack of participation. However, this did not stop the supervisees' high attendance at the groups!

CONCLUSION

Supervision in the nursing profession appears to be varied in both theoretical frameworks and application in practice. The historical aspect of nursing cultures, especially the hierarchical structures, does appear to negate the concepts of support and critical reflection in action. That said, there have been some traces of success within nursing supervision, not least the mentorship system for student nurses. Preceptorship does not, on the whole, appear to have had the same success, although the literature does suggest that, where it is implemented, the benefits are evident. Clinical supervision is still in its infancy, especially in the context of adult nursing, where there seems to be a general lack of confidence and knowledge to take this concept further. To promote supervision strategies in busy areas needs much thought and preparation. Raising nurses' awareness of the concept of supervision and its relevance to practice is crucial prior to any discussions on its implementation. One should also be cautious of the dangers of setting unrealistic expectations for what clinical supervision can deliver. It is not a panacea for all the ills of nursing.

Clear, well-structured frameworks and protocols for action must be developed by the clinical practitioners themselves. That said, the support from managers is essential to help take the project forward with confidence and success. In-depth education is needed by all the practitioners involved in supervision. As is evidenced by this study, although preparation was felt to be adequate at the outset of the work, on careful evaluation this preparation was not sufficient.

Supporting nurses is essential for the work they do. The physical and emotional demands of caring needs a forum to enable feelings about that care to be expressed and constructively discussed. The prime goal of nurses is to care for their patients to the optimum of their ability. If the participants in this study, through the process of supervision, perceive a reduction in their stress levels, an increase in their motivation and improvement in their communication, reflective and questioning skills, then surely the benefits of supervision cannot be ignored. That said, effective supervision in action is going to take time, but surely anything that is worthwhile is worth waiting and fighting for!

REFERENCES

Allanach, B. C. and Mowinski Jennings, B. (1990) Evaluating the effects of a nurse preceptor programme, *Journal of Advanced Nursing*, **15**, 22–8.

Bannister, D. and Fransella, F. (1977) *A Manual for Repertory Grid Technique*, Academic Press, London.

Bannister, D. and Fransella, F. (1986) *Inquiring Man: The Psychology of Personal Constructs*,. 3rd edition, Croom Helm, London.

Beail, N. (1985) *Repertory Grid Technique and Personal Constructs: Applications in Clinical and Educational Settings*, Croom Helm, London.

Bishop, V. (1994) *Clinical Supervision: A Report of the Trust Nurse Executives' Workshops*, NHS Executive HMSO, London.

Boud, D., Keogh, R. and Walker, D. (eds) (1985) *Reflection: Turning Experience into Learning*, Kogan Page, London.

Boyd, E. M. and Fales, A. W. (1983) Reflective learning: Key to learning from experience. *Journal of Humanistic Psychology*, **23**(2), 99–117.

Bulman, C. (1994) Exemplars of reflection: Other people can do it, why not you too? in Palmer, A., Burns, S. and Bulman, C. (eds) (1994) op. cit.

Burnard, P. (1988) Mentors: a supporting act. *Nursing Times*, **84**(46), 27–8.

Butterworth, T. (1992) Clinical supervision as an emerging idea in nursing, in Butterworth, T. and Faugier, J. (eds) (1992) op. cit.

Butterworth, T. and Faugier, J. (1992) (eds) *Clinical Supervision and Mentorship in Nursing*, Chapman & Hall, London

Cahill, H. A. (1996) A qualitative analysis of student nurses' experiences of mentorship. *Journal of Advanced Nursing*, **24**, 791–9.

Cameron-Jones, M. and O'Hara, P. (1996) Three decisions about nurse mentoring, *Journal of Nursing Management*, **4**, 225–30.

Darling, L. A. (1984) What do nurses want in a mentor? *Journal of Nursing Administration*, Oct., **14**(10), 42–4.

DoH (1989) *A Strategy for Nursing. A Report of the Steering Committee*, HMSO, London.

DoH (1993) *A Vision for the Future: The Nursing, Midwifery and Health Visiting*

Contribution to Health and Health Care, NHS Management Executive/HMSO, London.

DoH (1994) *Testing the Vision. A Report on the Progress in the First Year of A 'A Vision for the Future'*, HMSO, London.

Donovan, J. (1990). The concept and role of mentor, *Nurse Education Today*, **10**, 294–8.

ENB (1987) *Approval Process for Courses in Nursing, Midwifery and Health Visiting*, ENB, London.

ENB, (1988) *Institutional and Course Approval/Re-approval Process Information Required: Criteria and Guidelines*, ENB, London.

ENB (1989) *Preparation of Teachers, Practitioners/Teachers, Mentors and Supervisors in the Context of Project 2000*, ENB, London.

ENB (1993)A detailed study of the relationships between teaching, support, supervision and role modelling for students in clinical areas, within the context of Project 2000 courses, *Research Highlights No. 3*, ENB, London.

Earnshaw, G. J. (1995) Mentorship: the students' views. *Nurse Education Today*, **15**, 274–9.

Friedman, S. and Marr, J. (1995) A supervisory model of professional competence: A joint service/education initiative, *Nurse Education Today*, **15**, 239–44.

Furness General Hospital (1995) *Pilot Project on Clinical Supervision*, Furness Hospital Trust, Barrow-in-Furness, Cumbria.

Gibbs, G. (1988) *Learning by Doing: A Guide to Teaching and Learning Methods*, Further Education Unit, Oxford Polytechnic, Oxford, UK.

Hart, E., Bond, M. and Meyer, J. E. (1995) *Action Research For Health and Social Care: A Guide to Practice*, Open University Press, Buckingham.

Heron, J. (1990) *Helping the Client: A Creative Practical Guide*, Sage, London.

Jacka, K. and Lewin, D. (1987) *The Clinical Learning of Student Nurses*, Nursing Education Research Unit, King's College, University of London.

Johns, C. (1994) Guided reflection, in Palmer, A., Burns, S. and Bulman, C. (eds) (1994) op. cit.

Kelly, G. A. (1963) *A Theory of Personality*, Norton, New York.

Kohner, N. (ed.) (1994) *Clinical Supervision in Practice: Work from Nursing Development Units*, King's Fund Centre, London BEBC, Dorset, UK.

Kramer, M. (1974) *Reality Shock: Why Nurses Leave Nursing*, Mosby, St Louis.

Kurpious, D. J. Baker, R. and Thomas, I. D. (1977) *Supervision of Applied Training*, Greenwood Press, Westport, Connecticut.

Laurent, C. (1988) On hand to help, *Nursing Times*, **84**(46), 29–30.

Marrow, C. E. (1995) *Clinical Supervision in Action: Problems and Dilemmas*, Unpublished M.Phil. thesis, University College of St Martins, Lancaster.

Melia, K. M. (1987) *Learning and Working: The Occupational Socialization of Nurses*, Tavistock, London.

Meyer, J. E. (1993) New paradigm research in practice: The trials and tribulations of action research, *Journal of Advanced Nursing*, **18**, 1066–72.

Milne, A. A. (1928) *The House at Pooh Corner*, Chapter 1 in *The Oxford Dictionary of Quotations*, Oxford University Press, Oxford, UK.

Morrison, P. (1989) Nursing and caring: A personal construct theory study of some nurses' self perceptions. *Journal of Advanced Nursing*, **14**, 421–6.

Myrick, F. and Awrey, J. (1988) The effect of preceptorship on the clinical competency of Baccalaureate student nurses: A pilot study, *The Canadian Journal of Nursing Research* **20**(3), 29–43.

Ouellett, L. L. (1993) Relationship of a preceptorship experience to the views about nursing as a profession of Baccalaureate nursing students, *Nurse Education Today*, **13**, 16–23.

Palmer, I. (1983) From whence we came, in Chaska, N. L. (ed.) *The Nursing Profession: A Time to Speak*, McGraw-Hill, New York.

Palmer, A., Burns, S. and Bulman, C. (eds) (1994) *Reflective Practice in Nursing: The Growth of the Professional Practitioner*, Blackwell Scientific, London.

Platt-Koch, L. M. (1986) Clinical supervision for psychiatric nurses, *Journal of Psycho-Social Nursing*, January, **26**(1), 7–15.

Pollock, L. C (1986) An introduction to the use of repertory grid technique as a research method and clinical tool for psychiatric nurses. *Journal of Advanced Nursing*, **11**, 439–45.

Rawlinson, J. W (1995) Some reflections on the use of repertory grid technique in studies of nurses and social workers, *Journal of Advanced Nursing*, **21**, 334–9.

Ritter, S., Norman, I. J., Rentoul, L. and Bodley, D. (1996) A model of clinical supervision for nurses' short placements in mental health care settings, *Journal of Clinical Nursing*, **5**, 149–58.

Scheetz, L. J. (1989) Baccalaureate nursing student preceptorship programs and the development of clinical competence, *Journal of Nursing Education*, **28**, 29–35.

Schon, D. (1983) *The Reflective Practitioner*, Basic Books, HarperCollins, San Fransisco.

Shamian, J. and Lemieux, S. (1984) An evaluation of the preceptor model versus the formal teaching model, *Journal of Continuing Nurse Education*, **15**, 86–9.

Stewart, V. and Stewart, A. (1981) *Business Application of Repertory Grid*, McGraw-Hill, London.

UKCC (1992) *Scope of Professional Practice*, UKCC, London.

UKCC (1990) *The Report of the Post Registration Education and Practice Project*, UKCC, London.

Walsh, M. and Ford, P. (1989) *Nursing Rituals, Research and Rational Actions*, Butterworth Heinemann, London.

Clinical supervision in learning disabilities nursing

8

Sandy Bering, Ross Brocklehurst and Michelle Teasdale

'*I have tried to say that the field of mental retardation is, itself, unimportant. But it offers opportunities to examine the most important issues facing the human race. It isn't that secluding retarded people is wrong, but that secluding people is wrong. Or sterilising them. Or ending their life. In that sense, mental retardation is both the most trivial and the most important field.*'

(Blatt, 1987)

INTRODUCTION

Learning disabilities nursing is perhaps the most diverse and self-critical branch of the nursing profession. In the past, several practitioners have even questioned their continued value and role in effectively supporting people with learning disabilities and their carers. This followed a recognition that many of the traditional nursing models and support approaches were dysfunctional, and actually contributed to some of the negative experiences of individuals with learning disabilities who were inappropriately seen as 'sick' and a burden on society. As a result, a thorough national review of the potential contributions of specialist nurse practitioners in delivering effective and efficient services was undertaken by the Department of Health. This eventually led to a consensus agreement and statement supporting the retention of the learning disability nurse's specialist role, skills and knowledge base (Brown, 1994). Subsequent work through the 'Continuing the Commitment' Learning Disability Nursing Project has focused on highlighting the critical competencies of practitioners, examples of best practice and recommendations to maximize the impact of learning disabilities nursing practice (DoH, 1996).

The benefits of clinical supervision have been widely discussed, both as

it relates to the actual practice of individual nurses, and to the wider organizational care delivery setting, in providing the foundation of high quality
services to a range of clients. This assumption is common across all fields
of nursing and has been supported by the Position Statement on Clinical
Supervision for Nursing and Health Visiting (UKCC, 1996). A great deal
of literature now exists informing the reader of the practice and effects of
clinical supervision in other professional areas where care is delivered, but
there does appear to be a paucity of literature and evidence directly relating to nursing. This is even more apparent in the field of learning disability nursing where literature appears to be particularly thin on the ground.
Given the dramatic changes in recognized best practice in learning disabilities services highlighted in the recent national review exercises, this is very
surprising.

This chapter explores how clinical supervision is critical to the transformation of the outdated traditional learning disabilities nurse role, geared
to institutional models, to the current alternative community-focused
specialist practitioner who is operating within a primary care-led arena.
In order to illustrate these ideas, the important contextual issues of our
changing understanding of learning disabilities are initially described,
together with the evolution towards a community support model. There
then follows an exploration of the role and practice of clinical supervision
within a truly multi-disciplinary care delivery environment which seeks
valued outcomes for clients through enhancing health gain opportunities.
This leads to a discussion of the relationship with other key management,
training and personal development approaches necessary in effective organizations. Clearly, these ideas have relevance to other non-nursing staff
working in learning disabilities services who may come from a range of
professional backgrounds, although it is important to note the general
lack of an empirical base supporting the operation of clinical supervision
in all fields of nursing practice (Faugier, 1996).

UNDERSTANDING LEARNING DISABILITIES

People with learning disabilities want to be respected as equal, valued
members of society. They want to maintain or improve their lifestyles, and
to have opportunities to use the same services and facilities as anyone else.
Like everyone else, this includes the critical needs of access to a valued
home, financial security, work opportunities, experiences for personal
development and growth, leisure options, involvement in community life,
good primary and specialist health care, and opportunities to extend and
secure a broad range of relationships. Many people can lead an ordinary
valued life with minimum support, while others will need more intensive
or special support for differing periods of time.

However, having a disability in our society means that most people are also thought of as different in a negative way as our culture values being productive, skilled, attractive and affluent. For a variety of reasons that have little to do with individuals themselves, these attributes are rarely connected to people with learning disabilities. Rather, people have typically been wrongly perceived as 'incompetent', 'funny looking', 'children who never grow up', 'sick', or even 'dangerous'. As a result of these misperceptions, many people with learning disabilities have experienced a number of negative consequences. These have included low social status, rejection, segregation and congregation, loss of natural relationships, discontinuity, loss of control, deindividualization, material poverty and exclusion from valued social experiences. The history of professional services, including nursing, has often supported these myths by grouping people together, labelling them and creating 'specialist institutions' to keep them apart from people without disabilities.

Learning disabilities were once solely defined in terms of an individual's performance on intelligence ('cognitive') and adaptive behaviour tests. The results from these tests were then used to assign individuals to categories, such as borderline, mild, moderate, severe and profound. These labels were used to predict what individuals could not achieve and the disabilities were considered general and permanently fixed impairments.

Today it is widely recognized that this approach leads to inaccurate terms and unhelpful descriptions of individuals (for example, 'mental age' labels) as well as their support needs. The labels actually made us forget that each person had areas of normal capability that were developed or underdeveloped. The focus on reduced expectations has led to reduced positive and naturally valued experiences together with self-fulfilling negative vicious circles.

An individual's need for support will depend upon an interaction between the person's unique abilities, and the capacity of their physical and interpersonal world to encourage personal development and autonomy. This inevitably means that the type of help a person with learning disabilities will need will vary enormously and change over time, as well as across different situations. Development therefore can and does continue to occur throughout life and no behaviours can clearly define potential.

The definition of learning disabilities most commonly used for making decisions on providing services is 'individuals who have acquired their disabilities before or at birth, and during childhood and which result in reduced ability to understand new or complex information, and to cope independently'. Using this definition, it has been estimated that between 2 and 3 per cent of the UK population have a permanent or life-long condition referred to as a learning disability (DoH, 1995).

Particularly relevant to learning disabilities nursing, it is important to remember that individuals experience the same health problems as everyone else, but there are some conditions which are particularly associated with this condition and which warrant consideration for specialist additional support. These include epilepsy, hearing and visual sensory impairments, communication problems, obesity, cardiovascular and gastro-intestinal abnormalities, respiratory problems, impaired mobility, continence problems, mental health problems and Alzheimer's disease (particularly relevant to older people with Down's syndrome).

There is now a general recognition that people with learning disabilities will need extra help and improved opportunities to facilitate better health gains in line with the Health of the Nation strategies. Having the same needs does not mean that they can always be met in the same way as people without disabilities (DoH, 1998).

CHANGING SERVICE PRINCIPLES AND MODELS

Services for people with learning disabilities have been dramatically transformed over the past 25 years. Following the publication of the White Paper *Better Services for the Mentally Handicapped* (DHSS, 1971) and publications such as *An Ordinary Life* (King's Fund Centre, 1980), community services have steadily grown, and include a range of multidisciplinary teams and support networks serving people locally. This move has been accompanied by the transfer of resources from hospital-based settings to local communities, where the majority of people with learning disabilities have always lived. More recently, the agenda of the NHS and Community Care Act (DoH, 1990) has supported the emphasis of individual care planning within the 'support' framework. (See Table 8.1.)

At the heart of this philosophical shift is an acceptance of normalization principles (O'Brien and Tyne, 1981). This concept states that individuals are entitled to decide among options of living that everybody else has in the community. In particular, people should be supported to pursue lifestyles of their choosing that enhance their status.

Table 8.1 Emerging shifts in thinking in suporting people

Old	New
Focus on the individual's limitations	Focus on environmental constraints and capacity searching
Community readiness programmes	Guaranteed access underpinned by adequate support
Diagnostic-prescription approaches	Choice-based approaches
Separate services	Integrated settings
Emphasis on formal supports	Emphasis on informal support

A big part of the job of all effective professionals, including learning disabilities nurses, is to understand how perceptions of people with disabilities are influenced, and then to support more valued social roles through choosing status-enhancing supports, experiences, learning strategies and environments. The success of these approaches is judged by their outcomes for individuals, in terms of promoting positive relationships, personal behaviours, individual characteristics and roles that a community will value in a person.

Critical to this new approach is remembering that just because a person has a negatively-valued characteristic does not mean that we are justified in isolating him or her from valued community life experiences. Also, services that are offered should attempt to balance personal characteristics which are seen negatively with others that are clearly seen as positive. This includes supporting individual rather than group-based lifestyles, building on what each person can do and is interested in, making use of valued community settings, arranging ongoing respectful interaction, enhancing people's appearance, developing normal and predictable rhythms and routines, and developing wider networks of relationships.

Within this context, the nature of learning disabilities nursing has had to fundamentally re-orientate its focus and purpose, with previous institutional models and settings being abandoned. The new focus is on helping individuals with learning disabilities to lead healthier, valued and more fulfilling lives in the community. The struggle for individual practitioners is to understand the real meaning of support, choice, control, quality of life, personal satisfaction and community inclusion.

Examples of how these principles can be used in practice, even when working with individuals with learning disabilities who present severe challenges to services, have been described in detail by a number of practitioners (Smull and Burke-Harrison, 1992; Lovett, 1996). At the core of these approaches is a recognition of the need to learn to listen more effectively and spend more time in planning positive futures for individuals by considering what is happening and why, and how it can be handled better, through reflective learning of past experiences. These principles clearly support the value and essential need for positive clinical supervision strategies to be in place for all practitioners to translate these theoretical principles into reality for individuals with disabilities and their carers.

THE ROLE OF THE LEARNING DISABILITIES NURSE

As services have developed along the lines described above, the contribution of nurse practitioners has gradually included two very distinct but linked roles. The specialist nurse's distinctive role has firmly focused on the goal of maintaining and improving the health of individuals with learning disabilities, by taking actions which:

- mitigate the effects of disability;
- achieve optimum health;
- facilitate access to and encourage involvement in local community life;
- increase personal competence and feelings of control;
- maximize choice;
- enhance the contribution of others involved formally or informally in the support of the person.

The recent elevation of the key role of detecting ill-health and identifying conditions which may compromise the health and well-being of people with learning disabilities has re-emphasized and reaffirmed the retention of the nurse title, whilst acknowledging the broader social environment in which this work occurs. The specific areas in which learning disabilities nurses are expected to demonstrate health promotion and intervention knowledge/skills include:

- developing the confidence of people to make healthier lifestyle choices;
- encouraging positive mental health;
- promoting positive sleep patterns;
- promoting the principles of good nutrition;
- encouraging a more active life and appropriate exercise;
- correct positioning to prevent sores and limb deformities which make the person physically uncomfortable;
- helping the person become continent;
- monitoring epilepsy;
- monitoring medication, especially anti-convulsants and tranquilizers;
- helping the person and others to change challenging behaviours;
- managing stress;
- promoting personal safety.

Often, this work involves helping other health service providers and key carers who may have lower expectations of the health of people with learning disabilities. Staff specialize in a range of settings and areas, including working with children, working as part of a challenging behaviour team, or focusing on health gain strategies.

The other role performed by nurses is a generic function shared with staff from other professional disciplines, whereby individual practitioners assume responsibility to ensure health and social supports for people are planned, co-ordinated and organized to lead to valued outcomes. This work has clearly blurred previous professional discipline boundaries, as it has become recognized that no single discipline encompasses sufficient knowledge and skill to meet effectively the needs of all people with learning disabilities. The focus has been on utilizing person-centred planning approaches (O'Brien and Lovett, 1994) to design, develop and deliver effective positive support packages. This work involves various forms of care-planning that allow practitioners to:

- spend time with an individual with disabilities they know and trust to assess their needs and aspirations, as well as the requirements of those around them;
- develop formulations as to the major reasons for any difficulties faced by the individual together with successful outcome criteria;
- determine a set of interventions that will help to resolve some of the critical problems;
- monitor the effectiveness of these interventions against the agreed target outcomes and general best practice service principles highlighted previously.

This work requires: an understanding of the roles of a variety of staff, communication styles that promote collaboration; an ability to provide core therapeutic interventions; and organizational skills to target and sequence the help provided. In addition, there are several recognized general characteristics of effective practitioners that support constructive working relationships which learning disabilities nurses and other professionals are seen to need in this role (Bernstein and Halaszyn, 1989):

- They are accountable for what they do (for example, acknowledging failures as well as successes and learning from inevitable mistakes or errors).
- They treat everyone with respect and common courtesy (for example, listening carefully, taking time to thank people when it is appropriate, to be polite even to those who are rude to them and to be polite to those with whom they disagree, returning telephone calls as quickly as possible).
- They do what they say they will do (for example, following through on commitments, explaining reasons openly for any problems and attempting to compensate for failures, being on time for appointments and meetings, and generally being reliable).
- They are proactive (for example, focusing efforts on anticipating and solving problems, emphasizing strengths and building on the positives).
- They check their facts (for example, avoiding reliance on gossip and routinely obtaining information from several different sources before adopting a position).

Examples of how these roles are now being defined in current job and personal specifications for community learning disability nurses is given in Figures 8.1 and 8.2.

Within this context, leadership of multi-disciplinary teams within which learning disability nurses operate has increasingly been defined by compe-

Job Specification – G Grade Community Learning Disabilities Nurse

a) **Clinical Responsibility**
 1. To accept referrals of individuals and their carers as allocated through the intake process by the Service Head and/or Team Co-ordinator.
 2. To visit clients in order to initiate care plans (i.e. assessment, planning, implementation and evaluation)
 3. To provide a clinical advisory service on request to all agencies involved in health/social care support for people with learning disabilities.
 4. To organize own workload and work schedules.
 5. To plan, develop and maintain clinics.
 6. To visit individuals and carers in their own home or day settings as indicated in accordance with the programme of care.
 7. To manage the referrals, including liaison with referrers and GPs.

b) **Communication/Liaison**
 1. To organize and chair regular weekly staff meetings and other meetings as appropriate.
 2. To maintain systematic clinical and professional records as required by the service.
 3. To provide statistical information as required by the Trust.
 4. To ensure effective communication between health, social services and voluntary sector agency staff, and co-ordination of other services as appropriate.
 5. To participate in the relevant clinical, staff and professional meetings, as advised by the Service Head and/or Team Co-ordinator.
 6. To ensure interprofessional communications by regular liaison, case conferences, clinical reviews and reports as required.
 7. To develop complex care packages in conjunction with the Local Authority Care Managers.

c) **Managerial and Professional**
 1. To be responsible for the supervision and monitoring of caseloads for assistants and other staff, and organization of stays in the short-term care unit.
 2. To support students.
 3. To act in the absence of the Team Co-ordinator for the Community Support Team and to act across in the absence of colleagues.
 4. To observe and maintain agreed Trust policies and procedures.
 5. To be aware and maintain agreed Trust policies and procedures.
 6. To be fully aware of the responsibilities under the Health and Safety at Work policy and to ensure that other staff similarly comply.
 7. To inform the Service Head and/or Team Co-ordinator of other matters which might affect policy decisions.
 8. To co-operate with senior staff for the learning disabilities service in investigating complaints and mishaps within the Trust's service.
 9. To participate in Personal Development Planning Reviews and in-service training.
 10. To control drugs and equipment in the community according to the district policy.
 11. To institute and carry out research projects.
 12. To ensure a high level of ethical conduct in the learning disabilities service.

13. To undertake any duties as may be delegated by the Service Head.

d) **Training/Personnel**
1. To supervise and participate in the training of student staff and assistants within the community in clinical and organizational aspects.
2. To assess and evaluate the progress of students and assistants and report the same to the Service Head and relevant tutors concerned.
3. To keep up-to-date with current information and changes in topics relevant to the service.
4. To introduce new staff members to their duties.
5. To be an advisor on clinical support to other health and social care staff, and assist in the identification of staff training needs.
6. To facilitate the education of clients, relatives and other agencies concerned with provision of learning disability services in the community, through involvement in the Multi-Agency Joint Training Initiative.
7. To be involved in the development of training/information resources for staff in the area of learning disabilities and related difficulties.

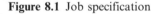

Figure 8.1 Job specification

tence in these qualities, as opposed to professional discipline and seniority. This is in stark contrast to the past reliance on clear professional hierarchies and rules governing professional practice. Today's mainly community-focused roles require learning disabilities nurses to stand back to assess and evaluate clinical situations on a more independent basis. This offers many opportunities for the development of truly individualized and innovative person-centred clinical practice. However, the work is inevitably far more demanding as the safety of past professional and institutional boundaries are gradually lost. Clinical supervision becomes critical to improve and ensure the quality of care provided by staff delivering both professional cross-disciplinary and specialist learning disability services.

The diversity of situations in which learning disabilities nursing is practised reflects a dilemma whereby the individual practitioner is able to operate within a complex yet dynamic arena. Lines of responsibility and accountability in these areas are constantly under review and often subject to rapid changes based on the varying competencies of leaders and staff. This dynamic focus often results in a unique transdisciplinary method of working, still in its infancy in other branches of nursing. Work in such an area is determined by the abilities, knowledge and personal characteristics of individual practitioners rather than traditional and inadequate professional discipline boundaries. This enables a greater exploitation of skill mix considerations, with practitioners recruited on the basis of their ability to deliver services sensitive to the needs of the service and the introduction of single 'one stop' intake assessments to screen work prior to its allocation to individual practitioners. Learning disabilities nurses need to develop as individual professionals who can integrate a broad spectrum of

Personal Specification

Post: G Grade Community Learning Disability Nurse

Essential Experience
1. Two years experience of working with people with learning disabilities and complex needs.
2. Two years experience of working in a leadership role accepting responsibility and directing others.
3. Experience of supervising staff both formally and informally.
4. Experience of working with people who are emotionally and physically challenging.
5. Experiences of accessing need/organizing and implementing care plans.
6. Experience of managing a budget.
7. Experience of close liaison with other professionals and agencies.
8. Experience of record keeping and monitoring.

Essential Knowledge
1. Legislation concerning medication.
2. The role medication plays in managing behaviour and side-effects.
3. Awareness of the needs of staff.
4. Innovative service models to support clients and families.

Essential Personal Characteristics
1. Ability to work in a highly pressured and structured setting.
2. To remain calm under pressure.
3. Empathy with the needs and experience of service users.
4. Diplomatic approach to needs and experiences of care.

Figure 8.2 Personal specification

knowledge into their interactions with people with disabilities and the community generally.

The experience of nurses working within the field of learning disabilities can reveal lessons and potential examples for other nursing care specialities within primary care-led NHS settings. The focus in this arena is the need for rapid accommodation to new client demands, where models of care delivery are directly constructed around the needs of individuals. One important development within this area is the introduction of alternative professional support structures by multi-disciplinary service managers to assist practitioners to adapt to a rapidly changing care setting. This includes the practice of how clinical supervision is organized.

THE CONTEXT FOR CLINICAL SUPERVISION

'For about a minute, Thomas and I are alone as he weeps in his chair. His tears are rolling down his face as his open eyes stare blankly towards me. He appears to be inconsolable in his misery and it is impossible not to feel pain and sorrow for this frightened little human being. Like his parents, I could not tell if Thomas was aware of my presence. He is blind, deaf, brain damaged, his limbs are useless from his cerebral palsy, and he is epileptic. It is hard to envisage Thomas's world.' (*The Guardian*, 3 February 1996)

This vivid description captures some of the critical issues facing learning disabilities practitioners. Society's view on disability continues to convey the impression that, according to the definition of imperfection and the inability of interventions to make individuals perfect, these people are less valuable that others. In fact, the inevitable consequence of this perspective is that individuals with learning disabilities, who are not ill and therefore cannot be cured, have a quality of life which is less than others, and even have less right to exist through the introduction of life-saving operations.

One critical aspect of clinical supervision in learning disabilities is to explore the ethical issues arising from judgements about perceived quality of life experiences. It is vital for an effective practitioner to have opportunities to consider their personal perspectives on these moral uncertainties. There are numerous examples of individuals with significant disabilities who challenge our assumptions about intelligence, through their use of a range of augmentative communication techniques which facilitate our conversations with them. These include the physicist Stephen Hawkins and the author Christy Nolan who at one time would have been described in terms similar to the extract from *The Guardian*. How is such diversity to be respected? When work is planned, practitioners should consider how value perceptions influence the clinical work undertaken. The changing pattern of thinking from making people 'ready' to live in the community and somehow earning these rights through passing competency and performance tests, towards the creation of a support framework where individuals are guaranteed access as citizens, fundamentally challenges the traditional rationale of many people entering the helping professions. Clearly, this move to a more equal partnership approach is challenging and can be threatening, especially to experienced practitioners who may be used to being in control.

Increased immersion in the community support role has also challenged the simplistic understanding of terms such as 'independence' and 'choice'. Practitioners often need opportunities to consider that there is no such thing as a risk-free life, as risk is relative and has a context. Too often clinical interventions focus on how people can be safe, before we look at what they require to be happy (Smull, 1995). This may necessitate a fundamental shift in professional thinking.

An ecological or holistic perspective provides an overall theoretical framework for the range of support packages individuals with learning disabilities require (Bronfenbrenner, 1979). Rather than seeing behaviour as either caused by some internal drives or a mechanistic response to external events, this framework views the ways in which people and communities act as resulting from the complex interplay of multiple factors that impinge on their lives. Clinical supervision may offer an opportunity to refine this model and consider three possible avenues of intervention:

- changing the person;
- changing the environment;
- changing societal attitudes and expectations.

This is in sharp contrast to traditional service responses which focus most of their efforts on changing the person. This clearly brings the practitioner directly in contact with social care issues such as where people live, whom they live with, what they do and any changes which may be necessary to secure the person's health and well-being.

Empowerment and self-determination are currently buzz words within most organizations. Clinical supervision can assist individual practitioners in developing the nine competencies identified for professionals to master in transforming their role to truely support and empowerment (Knoll and Racino, 1994):

1. an ability and commitment to identify strengths in people and groups;
2. a genuine respect for diverse perspectives and lifestyles;
3. a capacity to listen and reflect;
4. an ability to subordinate one's own ego (to put one's self aside in the interest of the group);
5. skill and creativity in helping people become more aware and confident of their own abilities;
6. appreciation of when to step back, and the ability to help the individual or group assume decision-making and action;
7. ability to analyse power relationships and help others to do so;
8. knowledge about how to gain access to information; and
9. ability to reflect on and criticize ongoing processes, including one's own role in these processes.

While this broader perspective is important as an organizing framework, clinical supervision can assist in ensuring activities remain firmly grounded on the experience of specific individuals. The concrete experience of individuals, rather than abstract goals or concepts, should be the focus of clinical supervision, and remain the constant measure of success or failure. This requires a recognition of the limits of clinical support, if there are overriding social or environmental constraints.

While the context is important, people with learning disabilities also need effective and at times specialized interventions. Individuals may need help to communicate, to manage emotional wounds, to cope with feelings of loss, to develop close and intimate relationships, to accept their disabilities, and physical health interventions. Clinical supervision should offer opportunities to develop competencies in these areas, or at least develop mechanisms for accessing clinical resources to meet identified needs and access direct practical advice or suggestions.

Practitioners also require opportunities within clinical supervision to acknowledge their own feeling of stress, and be able to discuss openly and honestly how individual pieces of work make them feel. This can extend to peer and other relationships.

THE SUPERVISION PROCESS

'Clinical supervision is a formal process of professional support and learning which enables individual practitioners to develop knowledge and competence, assume responsibility for their own practice and enhance client protection and safety of care in complex clinical settings.' (Fowler, 1996)

Within the learning disabilities arena, it is now widely recognized that clinical competence and credibility should determine the selection of a supervisor or mentor. It is likely that, given the blurring of discipline boundaries, no set criteria can be laid down to describe what or who makes a successful supervisor. As the maxim states 'it is possible to work 10 years and have either 10 years of experience or 1 year of experience 10 times'. The quality of supervision will depend on many factors, including the extent of the positive relationship between the supervisor and the supervisee.

The core purpose of clinical supervision in learning disabilities nursing is to ensure that actions take place in line with recognized standards of best practice, that these actions are monitored and evaluated within the context of available resources and the developed skills of staff. Given this, there are two major underpinning themes:

- Individual practitioners and supervisors meet to communicate, and resolve respective demands, make decisions and agree the objectives and tasks that produce a required level of service.
- Facilitation of direction, support and development of the individual worker, group or team, to adapt and resharpen their skills to meet new service demands.

Although flexibility should underline clinical supervision arrangements, it is suggested by the authors that the supervisor and practitioner should meet at least once each month for a formal, scheduled supervision session, lasting at least an hour in duration. Longer supervision will sometimes be needed, and access for informal discussions on matters that arise between formal sessions should also be made available. In addition, some form of mutual observation of clinical work should be regarded as essential, in order to ascertain accurate and constructive concrete feedback.

The following guidelines were developed by Community Care for Health (Chester and Halton Community NHS Trust, 1994) for the role of the supervisors who are providing clinical supervision. To:

- be accessible;
- ensure protected time for each learning disabilities nurse to lay out issues in his/her way;
- help the practitioner explore and clarify thinking, feeling and beliefs which underpin their practice;
- enable practitioners to identify and discuss critical incidents and/or stress-inducing aspects of their professional work;
- store experience, information and skills appropriately;
- challenge practice which is perceived as unethical, useless or incompetent;
- challenge personal and professional blindspots which are perceived in individuals or the group;
- be aware of the organizational contracts which they and the practitioners may have with the employer and client in terms of supervision;
- facilitate professional development;
- practise what is 'preached';
- make clear what is expected of staff professionally;
- treat practitioners with respect, even when there are disagreements;
- give practitioners regular, specific feedback about work performance;
- acknowledge that everyone has the right to be allowed to make mistakes and to learn from them;
- guarantee the right to confidentiality regarding supervision, particularly when examining constructive criticism.

The role of the practitioners, who are in receipt of clinical supervision, is to:

- identify practice issues with which help is needed and to ask for time to deal with these;
- become increasingly able to share these issues freely;
- contribute to reflective discussion;
- become more aware of the organizational contracts that exist with clients and the supervisor or supervision group;

- respond to feedback from the supervisor in a structured and professional manner;
- take complaints about the organization to the supervisor, not colleagues;
- behave as, and expect to be treated as, a professional, not a child;
- treat the supervisor with respect;
- give positive and corrective feedback on how supervision is working out;
- expect supervisor to have a professional relationship, not a close friendship.

CLINICAL SUPERVISION AND MANAGEMENT

The role of management in this specific area is highly complex, and it is suggested that the supervisory role is separated from the traditional management role. Supervision should be considered the right and responsibility of every learning disability nurse, as it has been previously identified by Ivey (1977) in relation to the practice of mental health nursing.

A number of other statutory factors have driven the need for a system of professional supervision. These being the NHS and Community Care Act 1990 and the Children's Act 1989, both of which created greater demands on the expertise of practitioners within the field of learning disability nursing. A number of nurses have found that the clinical supervision process enhances their nursing practice when properly conducted. Critchley (1987) notes that these nurses have their abilities refined as they are able to understand and describe more accurately, and assume less about, their own and their clients' behaviours and needs.

Managers may feel that clinical supervision is a threat to their management role, feeling they may loose authority or credibility. The issues of the blurring between supervision and control can emerge as distinctions, and similarities between these elements are often reflected upon. In particular, supervision may be an instrument whereby the health needs of staff are considered, the term health in this context being very broad. It may be possible to utilize the process and conduct of supervision in order to improve the overall level of management, as defensive management practices are relinquished.

The expression of the benefits accrued as part of this nurturing process is an essential part of the contracting and would therefore focus the commissioner's thinking to a view that clinical supervision is an integral part of the quality upkeep, and professional development of a service, with the inherent benefits for clients and their carers.

The observer of a service should be able to note the operation of clinical supervision within a learning disability team. Elements of the operationalization of clinical supervision should be transparent and the preceding features laid down as a framework for the audit of clinical supervision as an active element of practice. It should follow that the place of clinical supervision is explicitly identified by the Trust or other care provider within the Business Plan. The expectation of clinical supervision should be directly referenced within job descriptions, profiles and contracts of employment. A further significant step forward would be the necessity for all staff to embark on a programme that will enable them to develop as supervisors, in addition to demonstrating willingness to accept supervision.

An ongoing commitment to the evaluation and monitoring of supervision should be evident with clear performance indicators. This exercise could effectively be enhanced by user involvement in the ongoing evaluation and outcome monitoring process. The benefits of the process to the organization could also be exemplified by this action, as could indicators focusing on a reduction in sickness and absence levels and improved staff moral, as well as examples of increased service satisfaction by users.

CONCLUDING COMMENTS

The learning disability nursing project (DoH, 1995) set out its aims to:

1. examine, with key stakeholders, the range of skills of the learning disability nurse and to describe them;
2. identify best practice initiatives involving qualified nurses in this speciality;
3. provide advice on how learning disability nursing skills can be articulated to inform purchasers, providers and other interests concerned with the provision of services for people with learning disability.

Using the initial aim stated above, clinical supervision could be viewed as a method of allowing the practitioner to reflect on the content of nursing practice, thus allowing the practitioner to identify the skills of the learning disability nurse. An element of the supervisory process will be to allow the practitioner to describe the skills stated above. The practitioner, more importantly, will be able to estimate with some accuracy their own perceived level of skill in relation to each skill identified and formulate a development programme in collaboration with their supervisor. The definition of these skills will be more appropriately stated if they are referenced to strategies required to meet the client needs. This process will separate out those skills that may be inappropriate for the setting in which the practitioner is now engaged, and focus the practitioner's attention to the dynamic changes that have occurred around their practice. This is a very important factor as often individual practitioners will not have the opportunity to consider the total picture of their involvement with practice, as they may have been immersed in their own practice to such an extent that they may have been in ignorance of the broader operational changes that are impacting upon them and their clinical work. Essentially the process will enable the nurse to identify the skills required of them, and to be aware of the dynamics surrounding the application of these skills. A full description of these skills, their utilization and appropriate discourse will be essential to ensure that these skills are perceived to add value to the enterprise.

With reference to the second aim, identifying best practice initiatives, the nurse can exploit the clinical supervision process and examine reflectively the client's psycho-social, spiritual, economic and political background, their needs and the processes involved in delivering effective nursing care. A strategic analysis can be considered during supervision, the analytical perspective being the forms of interventions used and the reasons given for the selection of these interventions. The supervisory process could examine alternative strategies and estimations of the consequences related to these alternative interventions. The reaction of the nurse and client to the establishment and continuance of the clinical relationship may also deserve attention in order to allow insight into the interpersonal aspects of the nursing relationship.

Finally, the third aim of the project describes how learning disability nurses articulate their contribution to the provision of care. This activity will revolve around the ability of the profession to demonstrate that it is capable and has the ability to add value to providing care overall.

Learning disabilities is a field which has witnessed considerable positive changes over the past few years. This has been accompanied by an evolution in the role of learning disabilities nurses, with them becoming more responsive to the needs of people with learning disabilities, adapting to new working methods and settings. Clinical supervision is a critical issue which will be increasingly important in securing further improvements in services and opportunities, as it is directly concerned with enhancing clinical practice. If nurses are to improve on their current position, the issues addressed in this chapter will need to be more widely recognized.

REFERENCES

Bernstein, G. S. and Halaszyn, J. A. (1989) *Human Services? That Must Be So Rewarding*, Paul Brookes Publishing Co., Baltimore.

Blatt, B. (1987) *The Conquest of Mental Retardation*, Pro-Ed., Texas.

Bronfenbrenner, U. (1979) *The Ecology of Human Development*, Harvard University Press, Cambridge, MA.

Brown, J. (1994) *Analysis of Responses to the Consensus Statement on the Future of the Specialist Nurse Practitioner in Learning Disabilities*, University of York Department of Social Policy, York, UK.

Chester and Halton Community NHS Trust (1994) *Clinical Supervision: A Position Statement*, Community Health Care for Health, Runcorn, UK.

Critchley, D. L. (1987) Clinical supervision as a learning tool for therapists in milieu settings, *Journal of Psychosocial Nursing*, **25**(8), 18–22.

DHSS (1971) *Better Services for the Mentally Handicapped*, HMSO, London.

DoH (1989) *The Children's Act*. HMSO, London.

DoH (1990) *National Health Service and Community Care Act*, HMSO, London.

DoH (1993) *A Vision for the Future: Report of the Chief Nursing Officer*, HMSO, London.

DoH (1995) *Health of the Nation: A Strategy for People with Learning Disabilities*, HMSO, London.

DoH (1996) *Continuing the Commitment: The Report of the Learning Disability Nursing Project*, HMSO, London.

DoH (1998) *Signposts for Success*, HMSO, London.

Faugier, J. (1996) Clinical supervision in mental health nursing, in Sanford, T. and Gournay, K. (eds) *Perspectives in Mental Health Nursing*, Baillière Tindall, London.

Fowler, J. (1996) The organisation of clinical supervision within the nursing profession: a review of the literature, *Journal of Advanced Nursing*, **23**, 471–8.

Ivey, A. (1977) Foreword, in Houston, G., *Supervision and Counselling*, The Rochester Foundation, London.

King's Fund Centre (1980) *An Ordinary Life*, King's Fund Centre, London.

Knoll, J. A. and Racino, J. A. (1994) Field in search of a home – The need for support personnel to develop a distinct identity, in Bradley, J., Ashbough, J. W. and Blaney, B. C. (eds) *Creating Individual Supports for People with Development Disabilities: A Mandate for Change, Many Levels*, Paul Brookes Publishing Co., Baltimore.

Kohner, N. (ed.) (1994) *Clinical Supervision in Practice*, King's Fund Centre, London/BEBC, Dorset, UK.

Lovett, H. (1996) *Learning to Listen: Positive Approaches to People With Difficult Behaviour*, Paul Brookes Publishing Co., Baltimore.

Meyer, L. H., Peck, C. A. and Brown, L. (1991) *Critical Issues in the Lives of People With Severe Disabilities*, Paul Brookes Publishing Co., Baltimore.

O'Brien, J. and Lovett, H. (1994) Person-Centred Planning.

O'Brien, J. and Tyne, A. (1981) *The Principle of Normalisation*, CMH, London.

Smull, M. (1995) *Revisiting Choice*, unpublished paper.

Smull, M. and Burke-Harrison, K. (1992) *Supporting People with Severe Reputations in the Community*, National Association of State Directors of Developmental Disabilities Services, Inc., Virginia.

Swain, G. (1995) *Clinical Supervision the Principles and Process*, The Health Visitors Association, London.

The Guardian (1996), A Death for Thomas Kevin Toolis, 3 February, p. 18.

UKCC (1996) *Position Statement on Clinical Supervision for Nursing and Health Visiting*, UKCC, London.

9

Child protection: health visiting and supervision

Robert Nettleton

'...*we believe that, however experienced the practitioners might be, child abuse work is sufficiently complex and demanding as to require, invariably, good supervision.*'

(London Borough of Greenwich, 1987)

The development of supervision in nursing can be seen to be generated from a number of diverse influences, both within and outside the profession, as related by other contributors to this volume. However, the protection of children from parental mistreatment is a concern that has a particular impact. It is a concern voiced in the media, by the professions and by government, stimulated by notable incidents of what Dingwall, Eekelaar and Murray (1983) term 'agency failures': that is, by the deaths of abused children which have been subject to special inquiry reports or by apparently 'overzealous' intervention as in the case of Cleveland (DHSS, 1988a). Child abuse inquiries have stimulated considerable political and professional response. In particular, the Beckford report (London Borough of Brent, 1985) and the Carlile report (London Borough of Greenwich, 1987) link failures in the performance of the health visitors and social workers concerned, with inadequacies in the professional supervision provided by the field workers' superiors. In its critical account of the role of the health visitor, the Beckford report states that 'The aspect that has most troubled us has been the question of supervision'. The Senior Nurse told the panel of inquiry that the health visitors under her supervision 'were expected to recognize their own areas of weakness and of doubt about their responses to individual cases, and to approach her for guidance and assistance'. In contradistinction to this approach, the report states of supervision that, 'It must be proactive, and not just reactive' (London Borough of Brent, 1985, p. 143). In 1987 the Minister of State for Health asked the Standing Nursing and Midwifery Advisory

Committee (SNMAC) in the Department of Health and Social Security (DHSS) to form a working party:

> 'To produce guidance for senior nurses who in the course of their professional duties supervise, monitor and assist in training of health visitors and midwives in matters relating to child abuse including child sexual abuse.' (Press release)

The report produced, *Child Protection: Guidance for Nurses, Health Visitors and Midwives* (DHSS, 1988b; and subsequently DOH, 1997), takes into account the need for 'providing professional advice and for the supervision of staff' (p. 6) in a variety of specialisms and contexts. In terms of developing supervision this is of particular importance. The Carlile report (London Borough of Greenwich, 1987) shows scant regard for the particular context of health visiting. It places a strong emphasis upon the importance of supervision in child abuse (chapter 30). However, while its detailed discussion relates to the role of the social worker in the Carlile case, it states that supervision applies 'with like effect' to health visitors and their managers. This can be seen to be a misleading over-simplification of the case in what the Chairman of the SNMAC working party acknowledges to be a sensitive and complex area.

It is probably impossible to define 'supervision' too rigidly for all disciplines and settings, as each can be expected to have its own understandings and uses of such terms. 'Speaking a suitable language' requires that a language be learned, understood and used in a community of shared meaning and is a necessary component of a 'safe professional apparatus' (Butterworth, 1988) which is being demanded for dealing with child abuse. Munsen (1976) notes that supervision in social work is as old as the profession itself, but the term is used in a wide variety of ways. Parsloe and Hill (DHSS, 1978) have noted that social workers use the word supervision 'in a peculiar way'. On the grounds that it may be a fair assumption that each group in nursing uses the word 'supervision' in a relatively peculiar way, it may be helpful to focus on how supervision is understood in one grouping – that of health visiting.

'Supervision' has not been part of the language of health visiting, but this is not to say that supervision does not take place, is not recognized as a need, or is not valued in practice. The remainder of this chapter focuses upon field-work observation made by the author during a research project carried out in the late 1980s (Nettleton, 1991) which thus provides accounts of the practice of health visiting which may contribute to the development of supervision.

Part of the context of supervision in this domain are the varying 'ideologies of child abuse' (Parton, 1985) and the position of health visiting in this context (Dingwall *et al.*, 1983). Parton (1985) summarizes these ideol-

ogies as medical, traditional social welfare and radical social welfare ideologies. He follows Newberger and Bourne (1977) in suggesting two central
issues in constructing policies and practices towards families in crisis:
family autonomy versus coercive intervention and compassion versus
control. Social policy and professional response can be understood as
attempts to resolve the dilemmas represented by these polarities condi-
tioned by the ideologies of child abuse which carry most influence. These
themes emerge in the supervision of health visitors in the nature of the
health visitor inter-client relationship, professional autonomy, accountability and the role of management. Thus, differing perspectives concerning
the nature of child abuse have a bearing upon understanding the nature of
supervision. Put crudely, the performance of a health visitor may be
viewed in terms of her individual adequacy (or pathology), the environment or system in which she operates, or as being in need of liberation
from an oppressive hierarchical social structure.

FORMS OF SUPPORT AND SUPERVISION

Health visitors offer an unsolicited service to a largely well population
which includes all families where there are children under the age of five.
The SNMAC report recognizes that work with abused or neglected children will generally be only a part of the duties of community-based nurses
(DHSS, 1988a, p. 13). However, a number of studies indicate that dealing
with child abuse is anxiety-provoking or stressful for health visitors
(Bennett and Dauncey, 1986; Appleby, 1987; Gough and Hingley, 1988).
The main sources of support for dealing with child abuse take the form of
informal peer group support (for example, in the health visitors' office)
and managerial support. Appleby (1987) adds to these sources support
groups of which there are a number of accounts in the literature (Spicer,
1980; Vizard, 1983; Milne, Walker and Bamford, 1987; Richardson and
Dunn, 1987; Dare and Lansberry, 1988; Goldblatt, 1988).

Peer group support

An ethnographic study by the author confirmed that peer group support
was highly valued by health visitors in the settings studied (Nettleton,
1991). One health visitor, who felt good peer group support was vital,
related what she believed were the qualities of 'good' support:

> 'A trusting non-competitive group. You need to feel confident that if
> you disclose a weakness it is accepted by the group as normal. If you
> make mistakes, you are personally supported by the group, even if
> you're in the wrong. That is what you need. You haven't got to feel
> threatened by any one member.'

This health visitor's experience of peer group support was very positive. Her office developed a 'mutual appreciation society' which enabled them to cope better with very distressing situations. However, the office environment may not always be so supportive:

'I think it depends on how your colleagues are feeling. If they're feeling down you tend to feel a bit down as well with them, but if everyone's happy it's great, you know. You are affected by whoever is around when you're working.'

Another health visitor related a situation in which 'everyone was talking in the office but no-one could afford to listen, they had so much of their own anxiety to deal with'. She went on to observe that, like family, work colleagues are not so much chosen as thrust upon us. Supportive relationships do not just happen.

This can be appreciated from the history of primary health-care teams. McIntosh and Dingwall (1978) have pointed out the assumption made by middle managers in the 1970s that practice attachment and team work were synonymous, thus viewing difficulties as personal problems of individuals rather than as structural processes. Smith and Ames (1976) have also observed that the formation of a team does not necessarily equate with sharing responsibility for decisions in such a way as to be perceived as supportive.

Health visitors carry individual 'caseloads' although certain tasks are commonly shared. The extent to which professional identity is seen in individualistic, highly autonomous terms influences the capacity of shared decision-making. However, it has been noted that dealing with child abuse can induce a sense of isolation which can endanger good practice.

One group of health visitors endorsed the value to them of peer group support, but complained that 'there's no place on the stats form for it'. Later a health visitor pointed out that there was indeed a category for 'face-to-face liaison with colleagues'. It seems that not only do health visitors need to be given permission to engage in supportive activities, but they also need to be able to take permission for themselves.

It would seem that both personal and situational factors need to be taken into account. Talking with colleagues may raise anxiety as much as reduce it, for example, if the situation is seen as more dangerous, or solutions are proposed which are different to the one the health visitor would feel happy to pursue:

'You haven't got to feel threatened by any one member. It only takes one to be judgmental and uncommunicative ... It comes down to personal qualities, plus applying your health visiting skills to the group you work with. By that I mean identifying a concern weighing them down and giving them the opportunity to use you.'

In a research interview this health visitor, when asked, 'If you have one isolated or uncommunicative member, does it affect the group?', replied, 'Yes, but it doesn't stop the support – you get breakaway groups'. This illustrates the tendency towards what Smith and Ames (1976) term 'clique formation' which, while possibly functional for the group, makes the emergence of at least one 'professional isolate' probable. Thus, informal peer group support, while highly valued, has its limitations. The most supportive environment may not extend to all group members. The reduction of anxiety is not always desirable:

> 'We would positively say, "Well, I think you did a really good job."
> Mind ... we used to say you could probably rationalize anything.'

Dealing with child abuse can produce its own dynamics of isolation and paralysis. This is illustrated by an experienced health visitor who valued highly the support of her colleagues and her manager. Amongst the professional network – the social worker, the school, the community drug team, probation and the GP – this health visitor was isolated. 'I'll leave it to you', said the GP. He had indirectly communicated to her 'in code' certain diagnostic information concerning one family member which she felt added to the risk to the children. However, she did not feel able to share this with anyone. The other agencies disputed what action should or could be taken and 'meanwhile you are keeping an eye...'

> 'Jane [the mother] comes to see me – because I'm older than the social worker – she seems to accept me better ... I get forced into it by the mother – I'm trying to withdraw because I don't think its my role.
>
> I don't know what she'll do if he [the cohabitee] goes into prison ... you never know when she's telling the truth...'

The voluntary basis of the health visitor–client relationship characterized by a sense of continuing (rather than episodic) responsibility, with relatively little professional power, places the health visitor close to her client. While her anxieties are focused on risks to the children, who is the *de facto* client? The health visitor's isolation and vulnerability seem to mirror that of Jane. But who is the most 'powerful' and what is the power for? In this case, the health visitor is depleted and cut off from her usual supplies, seemingly unable to stem the flow, with no confidence that it reaches the children, the objects of her concern.

Managerial support

At the beginning of this chapter it was noted that the Beckford inquiry report advocated that health visitor managers should be proactive rather than reactive in the provision of supervision. On the other hand Dingwall *et al.* (1983) believe that the very existence of health visiting rests upon the voluntaristic nature of the health visitor–client relationship, an arm's length relationship with the state and weak management. They nonetheless believe that lack of public accountability is a problem which requires the strengthening of the supervisory powers of 'first-line managers'. However, as a Director of Nursing Services pointed out forcibly to the present writer, health visitors are considered 'first line managers in their own right'. Since the 1980s, the scope for middle managerial supervision has diminished further and clinical supervision has become increasingly differentiated from the managerial function. This does not diminish the responsibility of organizations for providing a framework within which policy and procedure are combined with the availability of supervisory relationships at a collegial level and in the form of specialist advice located within the multi-disciplinary framework of child protection work. Such specialist advice provided by senior nurses with responsibility for child protection has increasingly superseded that provided by nurse managers. While organizational structures have changed, and continue to change, the relational qualities of supervision at peer or senior colleague level are of enduring relevance and provide a perspective from which to evaluate whether organizations are fulfilling their responsibilities to practitioners and their clients. The ambiguity of health visitors towards support and supervision has been discussed. What are the qualities of senior nurses which are valued by health visitors, and which enable them to carry out their role?

Dingwall *et al.* (1983) believe that the principal determinants of service quality in health visiting are the individual conscience and skills of the field worker who makes the judgements which managers are obliged to trust.

One reason for this is that the work of the health visitor is 'invisible' and quality cannot be controlled by inspection of a tangible product or direct observational surveillance. A manager in post for about one year related this to the author:

'It's not enough just to know how the injury occurred or what action was taken – I need the whole situation. There is a distance between being involved as a health visitor and being a manager. The health visitor has got the whole picture in here [her head] of her contact with the family. To supervise health visiting I've got to have as much knowledge as I possibly can – otherwise its just, "Oh, fill in the review form, put them in the system, visit once a month". You could put that on a piece of paper – it's not really management. [Or supervision].'

Here is an indication of the skills required for supervision to do with enabling the health visitor to communicate her knowledge, and to assimilate it meaningfully. There is also the recognition of levels of supervisory activity. The manager acknowledges a dichotomy between a task-centred, rule-following approach and a more person-centred approach.

This vignette also indicates that there are various methods of communication which may be employed in the supervisory relationship. The 'system' refers to a monitoring system whereby children considered to be 'at risk' or of particular concern are reviewed regularly. The SNMAC Child Protection guidelines (DHSS, 1988b) indicate the value of a co-ordinating monitoring system. In the authority researched by the author, children who have been abused, who are considered at risk or who are of particular concern to health visitors can be placed in the system, activating the distribution of monitor forms at intervals determined by the field health visitor and her senior nurse. A senior nurse interviewed by the author described the purpose of the system:

> 'It is a method for ensuring that the families who have difficulties and children whom the health visitors (HVs) are concerned about are monitored on a regular basis – by the HV and the manager. It is not that the children themselves benefit directly, but it's for the benefit of the HV to discuss ideas of ways forward and draw on someone with greater experience than them. It's a way of HVs bringing forward cases – a forum for the HVs to discuss different problems without feeling they are failing by raising the issues. I think it is quite important – we are professionals in our own right and have to be seen to be managing our own caseloads and yet it can be difficult especially if you are not experienced, you can feel lost if you are not supported.'

The pattern of monitoring systems across the country is difficult to determine, not least due to changes in management structures. Such systems, although of value, have their limitations. Confusion can arise from terminology, such as 'at risk register'. It is easy to confuse a monitoring or supervisory tool for the Child Protection Register administered by the Social Services Department of the local authority under the auspices of an inter-agency Joint Child Protection Committee.

Secondly, too much should not be asked of such systems. They cannot themselves ensure the safety of children. The Beckford inquiry report (London Borough of Brent, 1985) notes that the health authority in which Jasmine Beckford died had such a 'Health Visitors' Concern' list.

Thirdly, such systems can be open to criticisms concerning the values they may embody. Who is being 'monitored' or 'supervised' by whom? Is it the child and parents or the health visitor? Recognition of this question is implicit in the senior nurse's account above.

This issue relates to a fourth limitation connected to the 'disease model' of prevention of child abuse. In this chapter, the focus is upon the process rather than the content of supervision. Suffice it to say, the 'risk factor' approach needs to be recognized explicitly as an exercise in value judgements. From the health visitor's perspective such systems are valued as a means to an end. The danger of a system becoming an end in itself is exemplified by the comment of a health visitor who said in the context of support and supervision that one might say things to a colleague which would not be said to a senior nurse because 'she would just say "write a report"'. Thus, rather than assisting the health visitor, systems may prove irksome. This is consistent with the observation by Smith and Ames (1976) of the conflict experienced by professionals working in bureaucratic organizations who may find them not conducive to professional support. They suggest that emphasis on bureaucratic procedures may correspond to a lack of professional resources for consultation. Thus, while the organization may be highly efficient at dealing with problems subject to administrative solutions, it may seem 'barren of expertise and moral sensitivity' when difficult, fateful decisions have to be made. It has been noted that a health visitor is powerfully placed to undermine an approach which does not win her support and appreciation, due to the 'invisible' nature of her work. More positively, when asked how she coped with a worrying situation the health visitor said:

'I talked to my senior nurse. I can phone her and off-load – not just write a report ... by telling someone else it makes you feel better ... and everyone is supportive in the office.'

One senior nurse interviewed by the author expressed the balance of responsibility in supervision:

'The spectre of a child dying from neglect or abuse must be every nursing manager's nightmare. One of the things I hope I have made reasonably clear is that I have the responsibility to give the support and know about the cases and help them [HVs] make decisions, but that they also have a responsibility to let me know because they have the responsibility of managing the caseloads. I have a responsibility to enquire and to be aware and we need to discuss and come to a mutual decision about how to proceed. I also need to be aware of the policy and procedures and ensure that they are adhered to.'

From this it can be seen that supervisory relationships cannot depend upon a simple concentration of power up an organizational hierarchy, but are characterized by mutual dependence and trust. The health visitor's access to a home rests on this voluntaristic basis and is thus highly (though not exclusively) relationship focused (Robinson, 1982); likewise senior nurses are obliged to trust field staff for their accounts of their activities. On the other hand, health visitors characteristically initiate and sustain relationships on the principle of the search for health needs, and senior nurses themselves can be proactive in providing supervision and support. This does not occur in a social and moral vacuum. All are subject to norms which indicate, often unclearly, the rights and duties of parents and professionals with respect to the needs of children. Policies, procedures, guidelines, systems, professional and organizational structures provide the visible normative context. They would seem to fulfil their normative function to the extent that they allow trust to be maintained on realistic foundations.

Dealing with conflict of opinion in decision-making illuminates the limitations of managerial supervision in health visiting and the qualities which facilitate effective supervision. When asked, 'Did you ever have a conflict with a manager as an experienced HV?' a health visitor compared her experience of two senior nurses:

> 'Well, Hilary just reacted. She was action-wise without really reflect-ing on it. But when I had Gill that was different – she was so superb – she would get you to the right point – she would help you to make a decision. You would come to a decision but if you were really stuck she would say, I think this. She was non-directive and you learned in the process, and sometimes there wasn't a decision and that was okay. Hilary is very clear thinking – she goes straight to the nub very quickly, but she doesn't always take you with her. It can feel to you like it's an arbitrary decision and you don't always learn from it – although it may well be a very good decision in itself.'

From the perspective of senior nurses in the author's research, direct conflict with field staff seemed minimal. This seemed to be achieved by heavy reliance on compromise:

> 'I can remember once when a health visitor wasn't happy with what I was saying ... I thought we would probably get the same outcome anyway. I think we agreed she [the HV] wouldn't go to the GP [about it], but give it another three days ... I think the health visitor is a professional and can make the decision as well as I.'

Does such a reliance upon compromise leave the door open to collusion? Responsibility for decision-making seems to be acknowledged to rest both with the individual field health visitor and with the senior nurse. This apparent contradiction seems to resolve itself in compromise. Thus, when asked: 'Where does the responsibility lie for taking initiative between the health visitor and the senior nurse?', a senior nurse said:

> 'In practice it is with the Senior Nurse, but you have got to make the climate right – you have got to make yourself accessible and accep-table to them – it's a dual responsibility.'

And later, when asked: 'Where does responsibility lie for decision making?' She answered:

> 'I think it's with me. When I was a health visitor I thought it was
> with me then.'

Thus, when this manager did over-rule and direct a member of staff she
described it as exceptional:

> 'It doesn't fit in with how I would usually deal with it. But I needed
> to take action on behalf of the child.'

The situation was also unusual because, to the senior nurse at least, the
line of action required was clear cut, whereas far more commonly situations lie in grey areas:

> 'What made the conflict "alright" was the relief that a long standing
> problem was coming to a head and her [the health visitor's] internal
> conflicts were over-ruled by me. She said to me, "What a relief".'

Given the importance of informal peer group support, one might expect a
manager to take this into account when difficulties arise. A senior nurse
described her role:

> 'I have long-term goals – to work quietly to resolve those sort of
> problems. I do not believe in confrontation unless absolutely neces-
> sary; it sometimes causes more problems. I feel I do have skills in
> manoeuvring people in ways that will sort things out – not dramatic
> – will cause the right result – it's over a longer period of time.
> There's one clinic with a lot of clashes, bickering about workloads,
> etc. I put in an HV who would be able to cope and I addressed the
> workload problems directly and they are working much better to-
> gether despite continuing workload stresses ... It's part of team
> building – the staff in a clinic pulling together in the same direction –
> not just individuals. I think it is very important because some work
> in quite isolated situations.'

Thus, although managerial and organizational structures change, there
remains a requirement for a culture in which formal and informal support
can be sustained so that practitioners can exercise their accountability for
work with the most vulnerable clients through supportive dialogue with
colleagues. The context in which supervision by a senior nurse for child
protection may be said to take place may typically include clinic meetings
with teams and one-to-one consultations on a planned basis or telephone
discussions, particularly in a crisis. Preparation for and attendance at
child protection case conferences and court proceedings also involve the
senior nurse. In addition to these formats and the use of monitoring
systems, there would seem to be scope for developing methods of communicating case-related material as a basis for reviewing practice through

supervision. In the author's own practice, genograms have proved useful in depicting complex family compositions and systemic questions, such as those in Neuman's (1982) systems model of nursing, in elucidating the patterns of resistance to change in chronic situations of concern. However, development of methods of supervision needs to take into account existing processes in order to be incorporated into a coherent model.

INTER-AGENCY ASPECTS OF SUPERVISION

A significant feature of the support and supervision of health visitors dealing with child abuse is in its inter-agency aspect. Peer group support can and does extend beyond the health visitor's office to supportive relationships with social workers and GPs.

> 'Sometimes talking with the social workers was very helpful to me – and having to understand the social worker's role so that you knew what sort of things you could off-load to them.'

The implementation of 'core groups' as advocated by the DHS (1988c) document *Working Together* formalizes the joint working of front-line workers in child protection cases. The author's experience suggests there is much to be gained from sharing consultancy skills across agencies and professions.

However, the differing places occupied by social service departments and health visitors in the child protection system predispose to certain tensions. When the former work under the principle of 'minimal necessary intervention' and the latter under the principle of 'the search for health needs' the stage is set for tensions to surface as in the following example.

The mother was aged 16 with an occasional co-habitee. She lived at several addresses, sometimes with friends and sometimes with her boyfriend and was occasionally homeless. The health visitor was very concerned that a young baby was not being adequately cared for at the level of feeding, clothing, protection from cold and general safety, especially with regard to the mother's violent co-habitee. The health visitor made considerable efforts to trace the mother and baby. Also her clinic attendance was minimal and she did not keep appointments to which she had agreed. The health visitor had placed the child's name on Child Observation System immediately and had also referred to Social Services:

> 'One of the worst things was the Social Services – I felt no one would believe me. I thought something was bound to happen sooner or later. I referred to social services but they kept saying, "What's the social work task?" I thought it was obvious – the baby was at risk and my concern was prevention. It was like I had to prove something

to them. Eventually the case was accepted and allocated when the baby was two months old. Then everything changed. I think partly it was that they got a new social worker – I know they had been understaffed. But she [the social worker] was really good. Before this they just sent a letter to her [the mother] and said they got no reply. Well, they wouldn't since she was moving about. I was out there asking in her friend's flat and asking the caretaker, "Have you seen this girl who looks like ... with a small baby?" At first he would say no but then when I said I was the HV and that I just wanted to let her know about the clinic so the baby could be weighed he said, "Oh yes, try that one".'

The case is taken up by the senior nurse:

'The mother disappeared for three weeks and when I got in touch with Social Services the senior social worker said "what more do you want me to do?" I said we should go to the police, but she disagreed. I felt it wouldn't have been harmful to the relationship [with the mother]. Because I didn't leave, she agreed that if the mother hadn't turned up after another 3 days I should phone the police. The HV had kept in touch with me. We had agreed she would try to find the mother and baby and she made every possible effort. I was concerned, one, for the safety of the child and, two, for the anxiety of the HV. So I decided I should take some responsibility. The social worker was quite happy to let us shoulder the responsibility without accepting the responsibility herself because there was no evidence of actual harm to the child. We sometimes say "well what do you want – an injury?" That's the difference between us – we are preventative, whereas the Social Services respond to a crisis, to an actual injury or to evidence of neglect. There is a difference between Social Services and us about where we feel they should come in and when they will do so. For example we make "information only" referrals for future use or to indicate that we have done what we could.'

This example indicates the supportive role of the senior nurse and some of the stresses particular to the position of the health visitor in the inter-agency system for protecting children at risk. Dingwall *et al.* (1983) describe this system as being underpinned by the liberal compromise, analogous to a separation of power in the state. Supervision in child protection needs to uphold the legitimate concerns of health visitors in the multi-agency arena, especially taking into account the deliberate avoidance of coercion in favour of principles of 'stimulating awareness' 'facilitating' and 'influencing' (CETHV, 1977), with respect to the health needs of children and policies which affect them. These principles simultaneously place health visitors closer to clients, allowing them to search for health needs, and make them vulnerable to shifting of responsibility by more distant child protection agencies. It is all too easy for the health visitor to mirror the apparent powerlessness of dangerous families to change, and their incipient violence to become reflected in inter-agency conflict. It is a key function of supervision to be aware of these processes, to identify their effects and to enable field staff to carry out their own role effectively in the inter-agency context.

ANALYSING SUPERVISION IN A CHANGING ENVIRONMENT

At a time when change can seem to be a rare constant in professional life, it would be unrealistic to propose models of supervision which did not take into account the policies which indicate the dynamics of change. Indeed, it is likely that supervision will to a greater or lesser extent be shaped by them. In the 1980s the Health Visitors' Association document *A Stitch in Time* (HVA, 1987) focused on the changes in management structure linked to the implementation of general management (DHSS, 1984) and the Community Nursing Review (DHSS, 1986). Concern was expressed for the provision of appropriate professional advice for practitioners. In contrast, in a more recent Health Visitors' Association publication, Swain (1995) distances clinical supervision from the managerial function. This is also the position articulated by the United Kingdom Central Council for Nursing, Midwifery and Health Visiting's position statement on clinical supervision (UKCC, 1996). In the context of the child protection work of community nurses, Parkinson (1992) asks 'Can managers provide both managerial and professional supervision?' to which her answer is essentially 'No'. However, the research upon which this chapter is based took place in the late 1980s at a time when these functions were largely combined. The Carlile inquiry report (London Borough of Greenwich, 1987) had stated emphatically that 'Consultation may conveniently be used to supplement, but never to replace [professional and managerial] supervision'. The members of the Commission believed it to be 'perfectly practicable for one person to perform the task of good manager and good supervisor to the same members of staff'. Certainly one of the challenges to health visitor managers at that time was the unrealistic expectation, that they could be sufficiently accessible and available to practitioners given the breadth of their role and the number of staff for which they were responsible. Contrary to the recommendations of the Community Nurse Review (DHSS, 1986), the 'span of control' of managers has widened increasingly and has been one factor in the endeavour to provide a systematic approach to meeting the need for focused support and supervision which is not derivative of the management function (Parkinson, 1992; Byrne, 1995).

However, more fundamental to the development of supervision is the supposed antithesis of supportive supervision on the one hand and managerial control on the other. The research undertaken bore witness to the tension between these polarities. The issue, however, is not merely academic but pertains to the nature of child protection practice itself: they parallel the issues of family autonomy versus coercive intervention and compassion versus control. Health visitors and school nurses, perhaps more than most if not all other workers in the field of child health and welfare, embrace the full spectrum which extend from child health promotion to child protection. Professional values have increasingly embraced challenges to a paternalistic basis for relationships with clients. For example, in a seminal speech Goodwin (1988) emphasized the voluntaristic nature of the health visitor–client relationship stating that an imperative for change is the recognition of the need for more participative and less directive relationships with clients. The Children Act of 1989 has underpinned partnership with families as a basis for child protection work and such values have found their way increasingly into professional policy and practice (Peall, 1992). However, the reality of child protection requires a confrontation of the vulnerability of children to those who, as adults, not withstanding the extent of their own needs and possible disadvantage, have power to protect or expose the vulnerable to harm.

What kind of partnership is it which allows health visitors access to the world of families where parenting may *not* be judged (*sic*) 'good enough' and in which the power to intervene is not denied? The qualitative research studies by Luker and Chalmers (1990) and Cowley (1991) provide grounded theories of how health visitors have developed practice skills and knowledge whereby they negotiate access not only to the physical home but to the life-world of clients and seek a shift from 'closed' to 'open awareness contexts' characterized by 'consonance' rather than 'dissonance'. These processes were also in evidence in the client *and* supervisory relationships related in the study. Managers were able to 'gain access' to the practice-world of practitioners not by using or denying their managerial authority but by consistently and unilaterally demonstrating a commitment to the welfare of children and their families in the provision of supportive supervision of staff. The 'invisibility' of family life/health visiting practice in any case inverts the formal power relations which may be supposed to characterize the relationships between health visitors and families, and managers and staff respectively. Those who may formally be taken to be in possession of the power of scrutiny and control are dependent on the trust which can only be earned but not assumed. While such trust is itself vulnerable, that is the hallmark of its authenticity.

None of the above is intended to argue for managerial supervision but to suggest that its limitations can partly be attributed to unrealistic expectations and more positively that the issue of power in health visitor–client relationships and in supervisory relationships is critical to the possibility, let alone the effectiveness, of supervisory relationships. The distancing of supervision from managerial functions does not dispose of the issue of power. This can be illuminated by an analysis of the UKCC's (1996) position statement on clinical supervision. The UKCC commends clinical supervision as a contribution to organizational effectiveness and identifies important 'links' between clinical supervision and management. It states, however:

> 'Clinical supervision is not a managerial control system. It is not, therefore:
>> the exercise of overt managerial responsibility or management supervision;
>> a system of formal individual performance review;
>> or hierarchical in nature.'

The analytic perspective which can be developed from the work of the social theorist and critic Michel Foucault is pertinent and illuminating. Foucault provides a penetrating critique of the human sciences understood as academic disciplines and practices of professional groups and institutions. His perspective is that the knowledge which constitutes human sciences flourishes or otherwise due to its correlation with power – hence his use of the term 'power-knowledge' (Gordon, 1980; Philp, 1985; Dzurec, 1989). A distinctive contribution of this conception is that power is integral to the generation as well as the suppression of knowledge, that is, the production of discourses, which can be understood as systems of possibility for knowledge. This is relatively easy to demonstrate in the field of child abuse over the short period of time from the 1960s when the 'syndrome' of the battered baby became recognized by paediatricians, through to the 1980s when, on the one hand, Child Sexual Abuse became a category for Child Protection Registers but, on the other, Satanic Abuse did not. Foucault suggests that within organizations and institutions power-knowledge is manifest through the exercise of 'disciplinary instruments'. Three overlapping disciplinary instruments are 'examination', 'normalizing judgement' and 'hierarchical observation'. By 'examination' the characteristics of one individual or group are compared with those of another known group. Thus, one may consider the benign example of the plotting of a baby's growth on a centile chart which serves to compare measurements with those of a normal population. It thus allows for 'normalizing judgement' about healthy babies and, of course, alerts professionals to failure to thrive, whether organic or otherwise. This is achieved by means of a system of 'hierarchical observation' through comprehensive child health surveillance aided by the technologies of computerized records and systems of payments to GPs. Disciplinary instruments are put into effect through the use of 'little punishments' to ensure conformity.

The fact that child health surveillance is now termed 'Child Health Promotion' (Hall, 1996) and that parents themselves keep their own child health records does not negate this critique for, to Foucault, disciplinary power is at its most effective when it is rendered invisible, not least by the complicity (in their own conformity) of those subject to it.

While this critique may have relevance to child protection work as such, it may also provide an analytic perspective upon the supervision of health visitors engaged in such work. This may be apparent in the context of managerial supervision and explain why it can intuitively be regarded as antithetical to professional or clinical supervision. Many practitioners may have experienced 'little (or not so little) punishments' from the hands of their superiors in an historically hierarchical profession with its structure of command and control, of policy and procedure. Thus the UKCC's denial that supervision is 'the exercise of overt managerial responsibility or managerial supervision; a system of formal individual performance review or hierarchical in nature' is a necessary reassurance. However, on further consideration, in the light of Foucault's work, a parallel may be drawn between these three features and the respective disciplinary instruments of examination, normalizing judgement and hierarchical observation. One might consider that the UKCC 'doth protest too much'.

The fact that managerial functions are separated from supervision does not guarantee that the disciplinary instruments with which they may be associated are thereby exorcized from the processes of clinical supervision. 'Self-management' may remove the need for a manager, but does so by locating the managing function with the managed. In the context of supervision this is captured well by the notion of the 'internal supervisor' whereby the practitioner monitors and regulates her/his own performance (Swain, 1995) exemplifying from a Foucauldian point of view the efficient use of disciplinary instruments.

It is not necessary to adopt Foucault's attitude of systematic suspicion to see in this analysis a corrective to the externalizing of the issue of power to 'management' or overly romantic views of partnership or collegiality. However, it is helpful to acknowledge that in child protection work it is important to face the abuse of power (over vulnerable clients and practitioners) and the necessity of the responsible use of power, which distinguishes *protection* from *paternalism*.

The idea of power-knowledge alerts practitioners that to hear the voice of vulnerable clients is to have the power to create knowledge of it or for it to be rendered silent: hence the relevance of the NSPCC's slogan 'Listening to Children'. The third edition of *Child Protection: Guidance for Senior Nurses, Health Visitors and Midwives and Their Managers* (DOH, 1997) identifies the centrality of clinical supervision which acknowledges the personal impact of child protection work as well as the need for a supportive framework to assist in the maintenance of professional accountability. The articulation of the skills, attitudes and knowledge required for supervision as a humane professionally-focused relationship represents a shift away from rather impersonal procedurally-oriented guidance of the first edition. Thus, one may be encouraged to believe that the 'invention' of clinical supervision allows for a fuller hearing to practitioners engaged in child protection work. However, questions remain about who hears and what can be done with the knowledge articulated in clinical supervision. One current feature of child protection work can be taken to illustrate the continuing importance of such questions. The research cited in this chapter suggests that much of the stress which health visitors experience in dealing with child abuse lies in situations which do not 'qualify' as 'child protection' but in which there is real concern for the welfare of children. These situations may be characterized by practitioners as 'grey areas' where 'you are left watching the pot, wondering when it will boil over'. In a situation where there are scarce resources and differing organizational priorities between, say, health and social services, the stress induced in practitioners is a political, ideological and managerial issue as well as a personal and professional one. The publication of *Child Protection: Messages from Research* (DOH, 1995) has highlighted the need to focus services on the needs of the most vulnerable families and not only those where abuse is alleged. Clinical supervision provides an opportunity for health visitors to articulate their work with such families, to identify the stresses and personal impact involved and to locate this work within a wider context of caseload priorities, development of practice and inter-agency working. This wider context is unlikely to be addressed unless the reality of practice is 'heard' by the organization. This seems to be taken into account by the *Guidance to Senior Nurses* (DOH, 1997) when it states:

> 'that clinical supervision in child protection is undertaken by the designated nurse or the named nurse, acting when necessary through colleagues. It includes reviewing with practitioners their *whole case load*, discussing cases of actual or suspected child abuse ... In addition, the impact on professionals working with families where children are at risk, or have been abused, should be considered'. (para 38, italics added)

If this approach is taken, then a mechanism is in place which enables child protection to be seen as continuous with the totality of health visiting practice. This might include the public health perspective by which health needs are not seen as merely properties of individuals but as arising within communities reflecting the social and environmental characteristics of the wider population. However, this assumes that senior nurses are part of a coherent organizational framework within which health visiting and related services are being developed as well as the inter-agency system responsible for child protection policy and practice. This assumption can be questioned, for as the centre of gravity for the organization and delivery of community nursing moves towards general medical practice, connections with this system as well as the wider health visiting network become more tenuous (Hiscock and Pearson, 1995).

Rather than simply viewing managerial control as something to be avoided, practitioners may want to consider how managerial influence can be won and utilized to provide an interface between the processes and products of supervision and the direction of organizational and practice development. Trayner (1994) has reported the dissonance between the views and values of community nurses and their managers during the 1990s. He utilizes Foucault's concept of power-knowledge to suggest that the norms and values of practitioners have been 'colonized' by inimical managerial values which disqualify the knowledge of practitioners. However, a feature of Foucault's conception of power which differs from conventional understandings is that while power relations are all pervasive they are always 'potentially unstable and potentially reversible' (Philp, 1985). This can be seen in the capacity of families or practitioners to control 'access' to their life-worlds by health visitors and supervisors respectively, so that the presumed direction of dependency in these relationships can be reversed. Thus, clinical supervision may offer the opportunity to 'colonize' the organization as the needs of vulnerable clients and the reality of practice are articulated, providing a means to fulfil the health visiting principle of 'influencing policies affecting health' (CETHV, 1977).

CONCLUSION

In the foregoing account of health visiting, child abuse has been identified as a most demanding aspect of professional practice. Child protection is defined in a normative framework, which is by no means fully consistent or static. Models of supervision need to take into account the particularities of the professional context, for example, the voluntaristic nature of health visitor–client relationship. In other settings common features of child protection work, such as inter-professional co-operation, have particular manifestations. For example, for the school nurse the relationship with teaching staff and their particular orientations are critical. In paediatric wards, dealing with parents gives rise to tensions when they may not be allowed to participate in the care of their children under the same conditions fostered by the ward's philosophy of care for children and families in general.

Professional accountability is brought into sharp relief by the glare of public attention upon the child protection worker. It highlights that aspirations to professional autonomy cannot safely be equated with isolation. A safe professional model for practice does not consist only of policies, procedures and management structures and systems, but these should underpin supportive supervisory relationships. Protection implies vulnerability. The anxiety of health visitors and others dealing with child abuse indicates the everyday reality of vulnerability. An appreciation of vulnerability also requires consideration of the reality of power in family, supervisory and managerial relationships. Perhaps vulnerability is a key to understanding how power can be harnessed or challenged to keep humane values central to the delivery of care *and* its organization and management. In the 1970s the social work profession grappled with its ambiguity about management and supervision for practitioners. One constructive suggestion emerging from research in that context was 'protection with autonomy' (DHSS, 1978). In this concept, autonomy is related to an implied interdependency. A model of child protection supervision needs to be sensitive enough to hear the voices of the most vulnerable, and to magnify them so that children and those who have their welfare closest to their hearts can be heard and protected.

REFERENCES

Appleby, F. M. (1987) Professional support and the role of support groups. *Health Visitor Manual*, **60**, 77–8.

Bennett, V. and Dauncey, J. (1986) Significant events for health visitors during practice, *Health Visitor*, April, **59**, 103–4.

Butterworth, C. A. (1988) *Breaking the Boundaries: New Endeavours in Community Nursing*, Inaugural lecture, May 1988, University of Manchester, Department of Nursing.

Byrne, C. (1995) A model for supervision, *Primary Health Care*, **5**(1), 21–2.

CETHV (1977) *An Investigation into the Principles of Health Visiting*, Council for the Education and Training Health Visiting, London.

Cowley, S. (1991) A symbolic awareness contest identified through a grounded theory study of health visiting, *Journal of Advanced Nursing*, **16**, 648–56.

Dare, J. and Lansberry, C. (1988) Health visitor support groups, *Health Visitor*, Feb., **61**, 41–2.

DHSS (1978) *Social Service Teams: The Practitioner's View* (P. Parsloe and M. Hill), HMSO, London.

DHSS (1984) *Health Services Management: Implementation of the NHS Management Report* (Griffiths Report), HMSO, London.

DHSS (1986) *Report of the Community Nursing Review: Neighbourhood Nursing – A Focus for Care*, HMSO, London.

DHSS (1988a) *Report of the Inquiry into Child Abuse in Cleveland* (Butler-Sloss Report), CMND 412, HMSO, London.

DHSS (1988b) *Child Protection: Guidance for Senior Nurses, Health Visitors and Midwives*, Standing Nursing and Midwifery Advisory Committee (SNMAC), HMSO, London.

DHSS (1988c) *Working Together: A Guide to Inter-agency Co-operation for the Protection of Children from Abuse.* HMSO, London.

Dingwall, R., Eekelaar, J. and Murray, T. (1983) *The Protection of Children: State Intervention in Family Life,* Basil Blackwell, Oxford.

DoH (1995) *Child Protection: Messages from Research,* HMSO, London.

DoH (1997) *Child Protection: Guidance for Senior Nurses, Health Visitors and Midwives and Their Managers,* 3rd edition, Report of the Standing Nursing and Midwifery Advisory Committee (SNMAC), HMSO, London.

Dzurec, L. C. (1989) The necessity for the evolution of multiple paradigms for nursing research: post-structuralist perspective, *Advances in Nursing Science,* **11**(4), 69–77.

Goldblatt, P. (1988) Connections and adaptations, *Health Visitor,* Sept., **61**(9), 273–4.

Goodwin, S. (1988) Whither Health Visiting? *Health Visitor,* Dec., **61**(12), 379–83.

Gordon, C. (ed.) (1980) *Power/Knowledge,* Pantheon, New York.

Gough, P. and Hingley, P. (1988) Combating the pressure, *Nursing Times* 13 Jan., **84**(2), 43–5.

Hall, D. (1996) *Health for All Children,* 3rd edition, Oxford University Press, Oxford.

Hiscock, J. and Pearson, M. (1995) *Perspectives on the Impact of GP Fundholding on Community Care and Child Protection,* The Health and Community Care Research Unit, University of Liverpool, Liverpool.

HVA (1987) *A Stitch in Time: Perspectives on Management Structures for Health Visitors and School Nurses,* Health Visitors' Association, London.

London Borough of Brent (1985) *A Child in Trust: The Report of the Panel of Inquiry into the Circumstances Surrounding the Death of Jasmine Beckford,* London Borough of Brent, London.

London Borough of Greenwich (1987) *A Child in Mind: Protection of Children in a Responsible Society. The Report of the Commission of Inquiry into the Circumstances Surrounding the Death of Kimberley Carlile,* London Borough of Greenwich, London.

Luker, K. A. and Chalmers, K. I. (1990) Gaining access to clients: The case of health visiting, *Journal of Advanced Nursing,* **15**, 74–82.

McIntosh, J. and Dingwall, R. (eds) (1978) *Readings in the Sociology of Nursing,* Churchill Livingstone, Edinburgh.

Milne, D., Walker, L. and Bamford, S. (1987) Professional coping, *Health Visitor,* Feb., **50** 49–50.

Munsen, C. E. (1976) Professional autonomy and social work supervision. *Journal of Education for Social Work,* Fall, **12**(3), 96–102.

Nettleton, R. J. (1991) *The Support and Supervision of Health Visitors Dealing with Child Abuse,* unpublished M.Sc. thesis, University of Manchester, Manchester.

Neuman, B. (1982) *The Neuman Systems Model: Application to Nursing Education and Practice,* Appleton Century Crofts, Norwalk, Conn.

Newberger, E. H. and Bourne, R. (1977) The medicalisation and legalisation of child abuse, in Eekalaar, J. M. and Katz (eds) *Family Violence: An International and Interdisciplinary Study* Butterworth, London.

Parkinson, J. (1992) Supervision versus control: Can managers provide both managerial and professional supervision? in Cloke, C. and Naish, J. (eds) *Key Issues in Child Protection for Health Visitors and Nurses* (Chapter 5), Longman, Harlow, UK.

Parton, N. (1985) *The Politics of Child Abuse*, Macmillan, London.

Peall, C. (1992) Partnership and professional power, in Cloke, C and Naish, J. (eds), op. cit., (Chapter 4).

Philp, M. (1985) Michel Foucault, in Skinner, Q. (ed.) *The Return of Grand Theory in the Human Sciences* (Chapter 4), Cambridge University Press, Cambridge.

Richardson, S. and Dunn, M. (1987) Coping with child abuse: Survival strategies for professionals, *Child Abuse Review*, Summer, **1**(6), 16.

Robinson, J. (1982) *An Evaluation of Health Visiting*, CETHV, London.

Smith, G. and Ames, J. (1976) Area teams in social work practice: A programme for research, *British Journal of Social Work*, **6**(1), 4–9.

Spicer, F. (1980) A support group for health visitors, *Health Visitor*, **53**(9), Sept., 377–9.

Swain, G. (1995) *Clinical Supervision: The Principles and Process*, Health Visitors' Association, London.

Trayner, M. (1994) The views and values of community nurses and their managers: research in progress – one person's pain, another person's vision, *Journal of Advanced Nursing*, **20**, 101–9.

UKCC (1996) *Position Statement on Clinical Supervision for Nursing and Health Visiting*, UKCC, London.

Vizard, E. (1983) Twenty months of Fridays – a support group for health visitors, *Health Visitor*, July, **56**, 255 –6.

10

The supervision of health visiting practice: a continuing agenda for debate

Sheila Twinn and Claire Johnson

INTRODUCTION

The process of clinical supervision, within the context of health visiting practice, has developed considerably since the first edition of this book. Much of this development has been influenced by the recognition of the significance of clinical supervision to high quality care by both government policy and professional and statutory bodies (DoH, 1993; Health Visitors' Association, 1995; UKCC, 1996). Although there is scarce empirical evidence to support this assumption, there appears little doubt that clinical supervision should contribute to client care. There is also considerable debate about the most effective approach to supervision. Swain (1995) describes clinical supervision as providing an opportunity to reflect on practice, whereas midwifery supervision is clearly associated with a competency-based approach to practice (Fish and Twinn, 1997). Faugier and Butterworth (1993, p. 9) cite the definition of supervision given by Butterworth as 'an exchange between practising professionals to enable the development of professional skills' which presents an interpretation midway between these two definitions of supervision.

In health visiting (as this specialist discipline in community health care nursing will be referred to in this chapter), the interpretation of supervision must also acknowledge the needs of both qualified practitioners and students. Although this position is not unique to health visiting, students entering this division of specialist practitioner education are required to achieve a second registrable qualification in an area of practice which is generally very different to that of their first registration. The demands made on students during the preparation for their new professional roles highlight the need for skilled supervision in the clinical setting. The Community Practice Teachers (CPT) who have this responsibility also assume a gate-keeping role in the process of admitting students for their second registration with the United Kingdom Central Council for Nursing, Midwifery and Health Visiting (UKCC). In addition CPTs, as practitioners, are recipients of the supervisory process. Because of these two different, but inter-related, approaches to supervision in health visiting practice, this chapter has three specific focuses. The first considers supervision in the context of health visiting education, the second considers the supervision of qualified practitioners drawing on different models of supervision and the final section of the chapter focuses on issues which we consider particularly significant to the development of supervision in health visiting practice.

SUPERVISION OF STUDENT HEALTH VISITORS

The student entering health visiting education is embarking upon a totally new area of practice. This is a different situation from other specialist practitioners in the community who are generally developing and expanding previously acquired nursing skills. Health visiting practice involves predominantly working with the well population, focusing on primary and secondary levels of prevention and the promotion of health. The focus on health promotion involves practitioners working at both a community and individual level (Cowley, 1996). The principles informing health visiting practice, originally developed in 1977, have been shown to be equally appropriate to current health visiting practice (Twinn and Cowley, 1992; Campbell et al., 1995). These principles, which require practitioners to search for health needs, stimulate an awareness of health, influence policies affecting health and facilitate health-enhancing activities, demonstrate a focus on the new public health movement and the implicit political dimension contained within health visiting practice (Twinn, 1991; Campbell, et al., 1995). The skills required to carry out this practice need to be developed during the health visiting component of the programme for specialist community nursing practice.

Health visiting practice has, however, been influenced by the changing structure of the National Health Service (NHS). The introduction of the purchaser–provider philosophy has necessitated practitioners in meeting the requirements of purchasers to ensure continuation of contracts for care (Buxton, 1996). This has contributed to the tendency for practice to focus on the more traditional interpretation of child health surveillance within health visiting practice. In addition, the emphasis within the current NHS culture on effectiveness and the measurement of outcomes measurement has contributed to practitioners focusing on the more tangible components of practice. These contrasting approaches to practice contribute to the complexity of care observed and experienced by students during their education and preparation for practice and has significant implications for clinical supervision.

The implementation of the report *The Future of Professional Practice: The Council's Standards for Education and Practice Following Registration* (UKCC, 1994) led to the introduction of a new curriculum for health visiting education in 1995. This change in the curriculum, the first since 1965, reduced the length of the programme from 51 to 32 weeks. The curriculum now consists of 50 per cent theory and 50 per cent practice, and is taught and assessed at first degree level. The requirement of a common core of one to two-thirds of shared modules with other community specialist practitioners is another significant change to the programme. Kelsey and Hollingdale (1996) argue that this presents both opportunities and challenges for students in the programme. They suggest a particular challenge is that of including theory specific to health visiting in the short time available on the programme. This challenge highlights the significance of the role of the CPT in the professional preparation of students, as the practice component of the programme now plays an even more essential role in providing opportunities for students to develop their competence in health visiting practice. Obviously an important part of this role is the supervision of the student while in clinical practice. An additional challenge for the CPT is the nature of health visiting practice which means that much of this time will be spent with the student practising without direct supervision.

The contribution of CPTs to student supervision

During the practice component of the course, the CPT is not only responsible for contributing to the student's theoretical knowledge of health visiting practice, but also for the integration of theory and practice and assessing the student's competence to practice. Hudson and Forrester (1996) argue the importance of the CPT in safeguarding the standards of specialist community nursing education and practice. The CPT, who is an experienced health visitor who has successfully completed the CPT course, has assumed greater responsibility for student preparation with the implementation of the new curriculum. The extent to which the CPT is adequately prepared for this role, as well as the adjustment of caseloads, will influence the quality of the supervision provided for students. Another important factor influencing the quality of supervision is the interpretation of practice adopted by the CPT and the extent to which the practicum is determined by this interpretation of practice.

The interpretation of practice adopted by the CPT will not only be influenced by demands of the practice setting, which may be determined by the requirements of purchaser, but also the philosophy of professional practice adopted by the CPT. This may be a philosophy restricted to a technical rationale approach focusing on technical skills and predetermined professional knowledge (Fish and Twinn, 1997). Alternatively the philosophy may encompass a broader, more complex definition of professional practice. This philosophy acknowledges the essential role of intuition and professional artistry in the professional judgements required of practitioners in making sense of unique practice settings (Twinn, 1991). The different philosophies and factors influencing the practice setting of the CPT will equally influence the learning environment provided for the student, which will in turn influence the quality of supervision.

The learning environment, however, will also be influenced by the quality of the practicum. Schon (1987) describes the practicum as a learning environment, which although resembling the practice world, is relatively free from the pressures or risks and distractions of the reality of practice, allowing the student to learn through actual practice in a protected environment. In order to achieve an effective practicum, the setting must obviously represent the essential features of practice. Although student learning may be inhibited if too may features of the real world of practice are omitted, this may also occur if too many of the practical constraints encountered in actual practice are experienced. Indeed, one of the difficulties of creating an effective practicum in the community is the difficulty experienced by CPTs in controlling the learning environment provided for the student. In part this is influenced by the caseload of the CPT and the extent to which adjustments can be made to provide the student with opportunity of exploring and understanding the fundamental principles of health visiting practice. Another important factor, however, is the extent to which the CPT can control the opportunities available for students to rehearse their practice in a partial or protected way. Studies suggest that, due to the nature of health visiting, practice students spend a considerable time practising without direct supervision (Fish *et al.*, 1990; White *et al.*, 1993), thereby limiting the opportunity for the CPT to observe and supervise the student's practice.

Another important factor influencing the learning environment is the quality of the CPT–student dialogue and the extent to which this enables the students to critique and reflect on practice. Fish and Twinn (1997) argue that the process of debriefing in student supervision is fundamental to fostering learning though professional practice. Studies, however, suggest that supervisors find effective debriefing particularly difficult, with much of the dialogue being descriptive, thereby limiting the quality of the supervisory process (Fish *et al.*, 1990; Fish and Purr, 1991). The difficulty of undertaking an effective debriefing dialogue in clinical supervision highlights the importance of the preparation of CPTs. Fish and Twinn (1997) argue that effective debriefing is essential to quality supervision and suggest a framework to enable supervisors and students to reflect on practice that has taken place. The framework, based on early work of Zeichner and Liston (1987), was developed from a small project which examined in detail student–tutor (CPT) debriefing discussions in the preparation of students for health visiting and teaching (Fish *et al.*, 1991).

A framework for the debriefing process in clinical supervision

The framework, referred to as the *strands of reflection*, has been developed from a philosophy of reflective practice and is based on four strands which provide a focus for thinking about the practice that has taken place (Fish and Twinn, 1997). The *factual strand* is generally descriptive and involves the student in providing a narrative of what happened in the practice situation. Although often quite difficult to recapture a complex situation, this strand involves three main kinds of detail: setting the scene, telling the story and pin-pointing critical incidents. The second focus of the framework, the *retrospective strand*, involves looking back over all the actions and activities that took place during the practice to identify patterns and possible new meanings from those reflections. This process encourages students to think about a range of perspectives of the practice as a whole.

The other two strands have been developed particularly to address the development of practice. The first of these, the *sub-stratum strand*, is concerned with discovering and exploring assumptions, value judgements and beliefs that provide the foundation for the ideas and events which emerge from the first two strands of the framework. This strand was developed to facilitate students in understanding the foundations of practice and to tolerate ideas that a range of views exist about activities in practice and that frequently there is no right answer. Discussions such as these allow real changes in practice to occur. The final strand is referred to as the *connective strand* and focuses on how both the theoretical and practical results from the three earlier strands might be adopted for use in future practice. The discussion resulting from this strand facilities students in developing plans for the next episode of practice.

The authors suggest this framework for reflection provides supervisors with a strategy to explore practice in a way which facilitates coaching the student and enabling them to learn though professional practice. Indeed a particular strength of the framework is that it provides a systematic method of investigating practice. The framework, however, requires a level of expertise as a method of debriefing and facilitating the development of practice. The use of the framework also raises some issues that require consideration in the process of student supervision, particularly when exploring the quality of the supervisory process.

Factors influencing the process of student supervision

These issues include factors which influence the supervisory process and are, therefore, implicit to the quality of the process of debriefing and coaching within the context of clinical supervision. The factors include not only the standard of practice demonstrated by the CPT, but also the CPT's interpretation of the assessor's role. Both of these factors have implications for the quality of the student–CPT relationship which is of prime importance to the quality of the supervisory process. In addition, the opportunity for reflecting on practice and the CPT's own experience of supervision will contribute to the quality of the clinical supervision provided for the student.

Swain (1995) argues that the relationship between the supervisor (CPT) and the supervisee (student) is key to the outcome of the process. She goes on to suggest that the interpersonal dynamics between the two individuals in the supervisory process are essential. Indeed, the quality of supervision depends on the ability of both parties to communicate openly and clearly. The one-to-one supervision process should allow for this activity by creating an atmosphere of professional intimacy where there is time and space to debate and discuss professional issues. The need, however, for ground rules to ensure the success of the relationship is identified by Kohner (1994). In the guidelines developed for supervision, she identifies the need for the content of supervision to be carefully defined, specifically in terms of which topics should and should not be included within supervision time. This is a particularly important issue for the supervision of health visitor students since research suggests that frequently the CPT becomes almost protective towards the student, particularly when the student is experiencing personal difficulties or stress whilst on the course (Twinn, 1989). The findings of this research also demonstrated the difficulties experienced by CPTs in providing constructive criticism to students, which is an essential role of supervision. Evidence such as this highlights once again the significance of the quality of communication between the CPT and student.

Schon (1987) also highlights the significance of communication within the supervisory process. He describes the situation of a *learning bind* as an episode when the student and supervisor fail to notice that they have missed each other's meaning in the interpretation of a practice situation. Schon suggests that the ability to escape from a learning bind depends not only on the supervisor's ability to reflect on the student–supervisor dialogue, but also acknowledging that it is not necessarily the student's fault in failing to grasp a learning point. This once more highlights the significance of both the relationship between the CPT and student and the setting of ground rules for supervision.

Learning binds, however, may also result from the standard and interpretation of practice adopted by the CPT. The standard of practice presented to the student will influence the opportunity for students to demonstrate, debate and critique strategies in practice. More importantly the standard of practice witnessed by the student may also influence the extent to which the CPT is adopted as a role model by the student. Authors such as Davies (1993) and Nelms *et al.* (1993) argue that role modelling is one of the most powerful methods of learning in the clinical setting. In a study by Dotan *et al.* (1986) specific factors were identified which influenced whether the clinical supervisor was seen as a role model by general nurses. Factors such as the extent to which the supervisor regarded teaching the student as important, the extent to which the supervisor's goals matched those of the student and the status of the supervisor amongst her professional colleagues and clients or patients were identified. Once again, the relationship between the student and the supervisor was highlighted as a significant factor, as indeed were the personality and the interpersonal skills of the supervisor. The attributes of the role model in the study by Dotan and her colleagues could be categorized into three major groups of traits. These traits were professional competence, a humanistic approach and power.

It is interesting that research in the health visiting education reflects similar findings (Twinn, 1989). In this study the data from the student cohort highlighted, in particular, the significance of the standards of professional practice demonstrated by the CPT and the personality of the CPT. Those CPTs identified as role models were described as enthusiastic, knowledgeable and interested. There was also a direct correlation between those students who perceived their CPT as a role model and those who considered that more time in the clinical practice setting would have been beneficial to their learning experience. The data obtained from the CPT cohort, although highlighting an air of resignation and inevitability, also demonstrated the feeling of power associated with the concept of role modelling. In part this was reflected in the intensity of their response to this question in the interview schedule (whether negative or positive). However, the power associated with the process was also related to the concern expressed by the CPTs that they should be considered a role model. There are, of course, particular implications of the concept of role modelling for the assessor's role also required of the CPT during clinical supervision.

The CPT, as the clinical supervisor, maintains responsibility for assessing the student's competence for practice in the clinical setting. Research suggests that this role is one of the least popular of clinical supervisors. In part this may be attributed to the responsibility associated with the role of failing a student. It also raises once more the issue of offering constructive criticism to students, which despite being fundamental to the process is another aspect of clinical supervision in which practitioners experience difficulty. Another issue which must be considered within this context is the extent to which the assessment of the student reflects the teaching and learning experience provided for the student. Although some CPTs acknowledge that the student's performance directly or indirectly reflects their input during the practicum, the concept of role modelling implicitly raises issues which require consideration by those involved generally in clinical supervision.

The need to be both expert practitioner and supervisor highlights the final factor for discussion in this section on the supervision of student health visitors. This factor relates to the CPT's personal experience of clinical supervision. Following the publication of the document *A Vision for the Future* (DoH, 1993) there is now a requirement for all practitioners to participate in the process of clinical supervision. This means that the CPT will also assume the role of supervisee in a supervisory relationship which may influence the methods adopted for student supervision. In addition, the contextual setting in which the CPT practises, in particular the trust's philosophy towards such activities as reflecting on practice, will influence the time generally available for student supervision. Finally the significance allocated to the professional responsibility of supervision by the employers of the CPT will influence the process. The process of supervision of qualified health visiting staff will therefore provide the focus for the next section of this chapter.

THE CLINICAL SUPERVISION OF QUALIFIED HEALTH VISITORS

There is a widely held view amongst practitioners that organizational changes within the NHS, particularly within the community setting, are creating structures which remove the traditional managerial supervision and professional advice available to practitioners (Jackson, 1995). However as commissioners reduce the managerial and professional advice component of contracts, nurses and health visitors in GP fund-holding practices will increasingly need to develop skills in clinical supervision, often in the capacity of team leaders. This development has coincided with the emergence of nurse practitioners, extending the range and scope of individual practice (UKCC, 1992) as well as the implementation of PREP (UKCC, 1994). Both of these developments clearly demonstrate the need for clinical supervision in the context of accountability for practice.

The increasing demands, particularly in health visiting, for a shift from universal to targeted provision of services (DoH, 1992; Audit Commission, 1994) and the trend towards role blurring within multi-disciplinary teams (Audit Commission, 1994) means that traditional mechanisms become obsolete and decision-making in clinical interventions potentially more complex. The expanding role of health visitors, as demonstrated in GP fund-holding practices has increased responsibilities without the recognition of the corresponding need for time to fulfill these demands. Indeed, a national survey undertaken by the Community Practitioners' and Health Visitors' Association (CPHVA) in 1994 revealed significant levels of stress amongst health visitors due to increasing workloads and a frequent lack of appropriate support since nearly 40 per cent of managers had no health visiting background (Health Visitors' Association, 1995).

These levels of stress and increased workloads result in part from role expansion and the increase in multi-disciplinary and multi-agency work, with the consequent complexity of skills required of health visitors. Working with a range of client groups identified by needs assessment such as drug users, homeless people, frail older people, young disabled people and vulnerable children and teenagers can create feelings of uncertainty and fear of a skills deficit for individual health visitors. These feelings are often amplified by the drive for marketing within the contracting process and lack of resources (Billings and Cowley, 1995). In addition, work in child protection is increasing, usually within a multi-agency framework. Although findings from a survey suggest that the majority of health visitors report access to specialist advice within a day (Health Visitors' Association, 1995), most child protection specialists provide support for at least 50–60 staff, as well as having training responsibilities. This allows little time to provide ongoing support and supervision for health visitors.

In this climate, there should be no question of the value of clinical supervision for health visitors. However, a commitment from employers is essential to ensure that the implementation is adequately resourced rather than merely a token gesture. As described earlier, the perception of clinical supervision by the nursing profession generally has been doubtful and confused (Butterworth et al., 1996). Bond and Holland (1994) describe fears about intrusion and 'policing' by managers at the heart of real concerns. Indeed, some implementation programmes fulfill this scepticism. Friedmans and Marr (1995) describe an initiative in an acute provider unit which has been designed to link clinical supervision to measures of professional competence and individual performance review.

In addition, the lack of empirical evidence to support the positive impact of clinical supervision on practice outcomes is seen as a major barrier to wholehearted acceptance of the concept (Fowler, 1996). Research is ongoing and already there are indicators that clinical supervision is viewed positively by practitioners and is particularly useful in facilitating reflection on practice and advancement of skills (Butterworth et al., 1996). However, the implementation of clinical supervision is at an early stage and further research over time will provide more evidence from which to judge the impact of clinical supervision on practice.

Nurses in other disciplines are currently exploring approaches to implementing clinical supervision and useful lessons can be learned from their experiences. Within these experiences reflective practice has played a significant role in the development of models of clinical supervision. Although a complex concept, with little empirical evidence to support the contribution to practice, reflective practice is considered by some authors as fundamental to the delivery of high quality care. The model of supervision described earlier in the chapter and that of the collegiate model developed by McCormack and Hopkins (1995) both draw on reflective practice as the underpinning philosophy. The collegiate model described by McCormack and Hopkins (1995) has resonance for many health visitors, particularly those working in professional isolation.

Although we provide an example of the process of debriefing in clinical supervision earlier in the chapter, more practical details of how to do clinical supervision are often useful to practitioners embarking on the implementation of the process. Titchen and Binnie (1995), although describing a model in the acute setting, provide valuable insight into the supervisor–supervisee relationship, relevant to both the one-to-one and group models experienced by health visitors. The authors characterize the relationship similar to that of academic supervision for doctoral students. They use this example to allay fears that supervision in this context means a formal monitoring process such as the industrial model frequently found on factory production lines. The work of Titchen and Binnie focuses on the 'expert' nurse facilitating the less experienced practitioner. This may seem initially more relevant to mentors and preceptors. However, health visiting teams and in particular primary health care teams, are composed of individuals with a variety of experience, knowledge and expertise so each individual may be an 'expert' in one scenario and a 'novice' in another. This approach produces opportunities for sharing knowledge and skills within the context of the formative component of Proctor's model of clinical supervision (1986). The authors conclude that the current lack of appropriate supervisors may call for the development of 'critical friendships' between peers in which there is commitment to observe, listen, question, share practical knowledge and to give constructive criticism.

Work to promote a developmental model of clinical supervision in health visiting, developed by Bond and Holland (1994), highlights a significant and continuing problem at the present stage of implementing clinical supervision, which is that of identifying suitable supervisors. Bond and Holland identify some key characteristics of effective supervisors and these include experience, having counselling or supervision training and considered to have specialist knowledge. These characteristics, interestingly, reflect those considered important in student supervision. The authors also highlight the need for specific qualities in the supervisee, such as a commitment to life-long learning, a willingness to consider personal values, qualities and skills and being prepared to reflect on relationships with clients. Indeed the UKCC acknowledges the importance of clinical supervision in assisting life-long learning throughout an individual's career (UKCC, 1996).

A recent training and implementation project undertaken in Manchester highlights the significance of these characteristics and many other important issues for clinical supervision in health visiting. We have used this project to provide a further example of the practical details of clinical supervision.

The process of developing clinical supervision in Manchester

The project was designed to involve health visitors with other community nursing staff in an awareness and training process to facilitate the implementation of clinical supervision. It is important to note that early discussions amongst practitioners revealed a strong consensus that increasing workloads had resulted in less time available to provide informal support for each other. The discussions also revealed that many health visitors felt that they had always undertaken some aspects of clinical supervision, particularly the 'debriefing' or restorative component (Proctor, 1986; Hawkins and Shoet, 1992). After the training programme and the initial evaluation process, however, all acknowledged that the formalizing and structuring process dramatically increased the effectiveness of their exchanges.

The training sessions covered a range of issues and provided opportunities for experiential learning. The content included an overview of the theory and literature, group function and dynamics, supervisor/facilitator skills and key issues in establishing supervision. The principles of reflective practice were used to focus debate and explore ethical dilemmas. Participants were provided with guidance on the practical aspects of setting up supervision, including formulating ground rules, format of sessions and evaluation methods (see Figure 10.1). The training process was facilitated by the University of Manchester Community Nursing Professional Unit in partnership with the Mancunian Community NHS Trust. The sessions were co-facilitated by senior nurses from the Trust and lecturers from the University. Four groups completed the training sessions provided by the Professional Unit in 1994 and 1995 and all practitioners who completed the training programme gave excellent feedback on the training experience and the implementation process in a group forum.

Piloting different models of clinical supervision

Following the training sessions, health visitors, along with other groups of nurses, selected models of supervision which they felt were most appropriate to their needs. These included one-to-one, group peer super-

---

Clinical supervision evaluation sheet

Date_____

N.B. The information on this form is anonymous. Items are not to be attributed to individual clients or families.

Duration of session

Number of members present

Number of agenda items

Number of members presenting items for discussion

Agenda items (e.g. child protection, inter-agency working, HV/client relationship)

1._____
2._____
3._____
4._____
5._____
6._____

Outcomes (action taken, e.g. further HV input, referral to other agency, reduce HV input, discussion with manager or advisor, consultation elsewhere)

1._____
2._____
3._____
4._____
5._____
6._____

Comments:

Figure 10.1 Clinical supervision evaluation sheet

vision and team supervision with an outside facilitator/supervisor from the same discipline. No specific mode of supervision was advocated. Individuals and groups adopted approaches which were appropriate to their unique situation. For example, some preferred highly structured formats, while others adopted a more informal approach. Reflective approaches to supervision were popular with practitioners using both one-to-one and group supervision. Models developed by Johns (1993) and Proctor (1986) were used by a number of participants since the majority wished to avoid a counselling model of supervision (Hawkins and Shoet, 1992).

To illustrate the different experiences of practitioners involved in clinical supervision we have used the health visitors' personal accounts of episodes which occurred during the supervision sessions of two of the pilot groups.

Episode I: The reflective mode in clinical supervision
'One session in our group clinical supervision clearly identified reflective supervision as being important in its own right.

I had brought a family from my caseload which had multiple problems and had received intensive health visiting input and referrals to other agencies.

I had come to a "deadlock" in my work with the family and had begun to feel that my input needed to be reviewed. As I presented the family to the group, there were plenty of suggestions for possible courses of action, some of which had already been tried. I began to realize that I did not want advice on this occasion, but needed to be listened to as I thought aloud. The end result was that I acknowledged, with the affirmation of the group, that I had probably done all that I could with the family for the present time and could now step back.

Had I not had this opportunity to discuss this family in a supportive way I may have withdrawn from the family and their problems without being able to acknowledge that they were at that time unable to "move on".

In retrospect, we as a group identified that it is OK just to listen reflectively in supervision without necessarily giving advice or direction, so enabling the supervisee to find her or his way.'

Episode II: The unexpected outcomes of clinical supervision
'Four health visitors were discussing drug abuse and the potential health and lifestyle risks to which even quite young children are exposed nowadays. One of the health visitors suddenly became upset as she realized for the first time how concerned she was about the future wellbeing of her young grandchildren.

The supervisor and two of the other three health visitors seemed to be comfortable with these feelings being exposed within the group, but the third health visitor blocked the discussion saying that she did not think the "upset" health visitor would want to be further embarrassed. However, once she had recovered from her surprise at her unexpected reaction, the "upset" health visitor found that this had been a useful experience. Becoming aware of her anxiety enabled her to analyse her response and come to terms with it.

It also gave her another insight into why clients react as they do sometimes to events in their lives and so was a positive aid to good practice.'

KEY ISSUES IDENTIFIED FROM THE CLINICAL SUPERVISION PROJECTS

The evaluation and review of the pilot projects were conducted in several ways with all the projects carrying out an on-going evaluation process. For example in one group all members completed individual reflective diaries after each session and used the material at the start of each session in order to follow up issues raised previously. This method provided an opportunity for each individual to reflect on issues raised after the session, rather than only those raised during the clinical supervision process and proved to be very constructive. A further example is provided by a team supervision group who evaluated the process in a discussion group with an external facilitator. Another carried out a similar process with a facilitator involved in their peer supervision group.

Indeed it emerged during the review process that health visitors had individual approaches to key areas of work such as problem-solving which they had not recognized before, despite working closely in teams. One group demonstrated a healthy tension in their various approaches to problem-solving (Figure 10.2) and in identifying the diversity in their approach were able to promote valuable debate and effective action planning. In facilitating the evaluation process with another group of health visitors it was possible to categorize the content of supervision sessions using the model of supervision developed by Proctor (1986) (Figure 10.3).

The process of evaluation and review of the projects identified several key themes which have implications for the implementation and maintenance of clinical supervision in the community setting. Indeed from the wealth of material generated during the feedback sessions of the pilot projects the following themes were identified using the principles of content and thematic analysis. (Polit and Hungler, 1995; Robson, 1996).

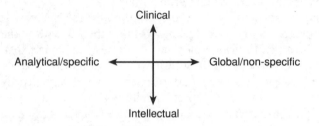

Figure 10.2 Approaches to problem-solving in group supervision

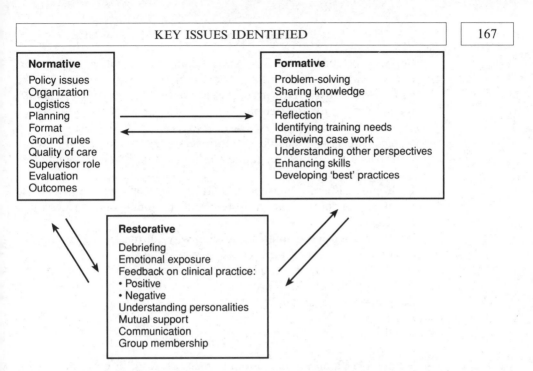

Normative

Policy issues
Organization
Logistics
Planning
Format
Ground rules
Quality of care
Supervisor role
Evaluation
Outcomes

Formative

Problem-solving
Sharing knowledge
Education
Reflection
Identifying training needs
Reviewing case work
Understanding other perspectives
Enhancing skills
Developing 'best' practices

Restorative

Debriefing
Emotional exposure
Feedback on clinical practice:
• Positive
• Negative
Understanding personalities
Mutual support
Communication
Group membership

Figure 10.3 Clinical supervision in practice: Application of Proctor's model (1986)

The themes could be categorized into the following areas:

- *Organizational*:
  - It is essential to make clinical supervision a priority at a organizational level
  - Time was identified as a crucial factor. The commitment of managers and staff is required so that clinical supervision time is not eroded by other service needs
  - Keeping clinical supervision going requires determination and enthusiasm, particularly when the workload is high
  - Staff shortages and overwork can threaten clinical supervision in the very circumstances where it is most vital
  - It is important to establish and review the ground rules
  - Participants in clinical supervision need to be prepared to adjust and adapt the process as experience highlights the need for change or modification.
- *Support*
  - Supervision was identified as a means of supporting practitioners in their work. Health visitors often work alone with clients, sometimes in stressful and difficult circumstances and all those involved recognized the value of support for practitioners

– Support for supervisors. For those taking on the role of supervisor, it is essential that a support mechanism is in place to provide the supervisor with their own supervision as well as provide a channel for accountability and action.

- *Improving practice*
  – Clinical supervision enables practitioners to be creative
  – It provides a forum to examine conflicts of approach to practice in a non-threatening way
  – It brings different perspectives to a problem by utilizing the resources of individuals arising from personal and professional experience
  – It provides an opportunity to develop ways of measuring the impact of clinical supervision on practice
  – By reviewing practice outcomes, clinical supervision enables practitioners to identify and disseminate 'best practice' therefore potentially improving the quality of care.

- *Content*
  – Child protection issues
  – Casework focus
  – Vulnerable families and groups such as drug users, those with chronic illness, those with life-threatening illness, isolated older people, young disabled people, homeless people, those in poverty, those in severe emotional crisis, those with mental health problems, families and individuals who are hard to engage
  – Barriers to effective team working. This may occur within the PHCT, at the primary/secondary care interface or within interagency working
  – Episodes/incidents stressful to the health visitor concerned
  – Sharing knowledge and engaging in critical debate about approaches to assessment, planning, intervention and evaluation.

- *Confidentiality and ethical issues*:
  – Risks of emotional exposure for practitioners
  – Risk of exposing poor practice
  – Conflicts between confidentiality and need for evaluation
  – Risks to the organization. This may include issues which have implications outside the supervision forum such as policy matters and unmet needs.

    The issues and themes arising in these major areas need to be fully debated by participants at the stage of setting the ground rules for clinical supervision so that each individual or group member understands the consequences of disclosure before such circumstances arise.

- *Team building*
  – The importance of involving all grades of staff. Increasingly this has

become relevant to all health visitors with the growth of skill-mix and multi-disciplinary teams. A general view emerging is that all those who deal directly with service users in the clinical setting need to be involved in clinical supervision at some level
- Improving communication and relationships between existing colleagues. This was seen as a clear and immediate advantage to those involved and was directly attributed to the process of engaging in clinical supervision
- Equity within the process: removing the effects of individual dominance. This highlights the importance of structure in the sessions and the need for skilled facilitation.

● *Training*
- The need for training for all staff involved: supervisors and supervisees. This is considered vital for successful implementation. The shortage of appropriately qualified and experienced trainers will remain an issue until expertise in this area is more readily available within nursing
- The need for knowledge and understanding to enrich the process and maximize the potential of clinical supervision. Many participants acknowledged the value of the training for supervision they had undertaken to their role as supervisees within a group, highlighting the need for supervisee training.

CONCLUSIONS: DEVELOPING CLINICAL SUPERVISION IN HEALTH VISITING PRACTICE

It is our belief that the issues identified above are very important to the success and development of clinical supervision in health visiting practice. Although the evidence from individuals and groups about the experience of clinical supervision in Manchester is both positive and encouraging, there remain a number of key areas which practitioners need to consider when thinking about clinical supervision. The first of these issues relates to the affect of clinical supervision on the quality of practice, in particular whether clinical supervision has a demonstrable impact on standards of practice which will benefit both the practitioner and service user. The lack of empirical evidence highlights the need for research into the effect of clinical supervision on the quality of care.

The need to provide appropriate training for all those involved in clinical supervision is another important issue. A key area of need appears to be in skills training to enhance and develop communication skills. Although interaction and communication skills are included in health visitor education, many participants were clear that these basic communication skills were insufficient and that more advanced skills training were essential such as in-depth work on group dynamics, team work and dealing with challenging situations, confrontation, giving feedback and skills of reflection. These skills and attributes appear to be essential in promoting the exchange between practising professionals within the context of clinical supervision advocated by Butterworth (1992). The skills are equally important whether using one-to-one or group models of supervision and in the supervision of student health visitors, particularly in enhancing the student–supervisor relationship. In addition, a considerable advantage to training programmes designed to deliver such skills is that these skills are of significant value in many areas of health visiting practice and therefore represent genuinely transferable skills which makes training widely applicable and cost effective.

The different models of supervision also emerged as an issue for consideration by practitioners. The significance of the interpretation of clinical supervision, particularly within a gate-keeping capacity, has been highlighted in the context of student supervision. For qualified practitioners, the NHSE at the Department of Health in England, in their circular on the implementation and evaluation of clinical supervision (DoH, 1995), has highlighted the requirement for national and local debate on the range and appropriateness of models of clinical supervision. The emphasis, however, must be on local issues and needs. Indeed, the UKCC Position Paper on clinical supervision (UKCC, 1996) argues against a prescriptive approach to implementation, effectively supporting a grass roots approach. This places the responsibility firmly on purchasers and providers to ensure that development and evaluation takes place at a local level. The responsibility on purchasers and providers is also demonstrated in the consultation exercise undertaken by the NHSE on the development of clinical supervision models (DoH, 1994) This highlights the need for an improved understanding of the cost benefits of clinical supervision between purchasers and providers. In addition, it is suggested that the identification of models of clinical supervision and exploration of implementation and evaluation would be of value to providers.

In our view these issues highlight the need for health visitors to build in evaluation strategies when implementing programmes of clinical supervision and take a lead in research investigating the effectiveness of the process. Health visitors are also ideally placed to be the prime movers in facilitating the development of clinical supervision in the multi-disciplinary setting of primary health care. It is this next phase of development which is perhaps the most significant if positive outcomes for service users are to be the primary focus of clinical supervision.

REFERENCES

Audit Commision (1994) *Seen But Not Heard: Co-ordinating Community Child Health and Social Services for Children in Need*, HMSO, London.

Billings, J. R. and Cowley, S. (1995) Approaches to commuity needs assessment: A literature review, *Journal of Advanced Nursing*, **22**, 721–30.

Bond, M. and Holland, S. (1994) Developmental supervision in health visiting, *Health Visitor*, **67**(11), 392–3.

Butterworth, T. (1992) Clinical supervision as an emerging idea in nursing, in Butterworth, T. amd Faugier, J. (eds) *Clinical Supervison and Mentorship in Nursing*, Chapman & Hall, London.

Butterworth, T., Bishop, V. and Carson, J. (1996) First steps towards evaluating clinical supervision in nursing, midwifery and health visiting. 1 Theory, policy and practice development: A review, *Journal of Clinical Nursing*, **5**(2), 127–32.

Buxton, V. (1996) Strength in diversity, *Nursing Times*, **92**(28), 63.

Campbell, F., Cowley, S. and Buttigieg, M. (1995) *Weights and Measures: Outcomes and Evaluation in Health Visiting*, Health Visitors' Association, London.

Cowley, S. (1996) Reflecting on the past; Preparing for the next century, *Health Visitor*, **69**(8), 313–16.

Davies. E. (1993) Clinical role modelling: Uncovering hidden knowledge, *Journal of Advanced Nursing*, **18**, 627–36.

DoH (1992) *The Health of the Nation: A Strategy for Health in England*, HMSO, London.

DoH (1993) *A Vision for the Future: The Nursing, Midwifery and Health Visiting Contribution to Health and Health Care*, HMSO, London.

DoH (1994) *Testing the Vision: A Report on Progress in the First Year of 'A Vision for the Future'*, HMSO, London.

DoH (1995) *A Vision for the Future: Report of the Consulation Exercise on Target Development in 'A Vision for the Future'*, HMSO, London.

Dotan, M., Krulik, T., Bergman, R., Eckerling, S. and Shatzman, H. (1986) Role models in nursing, *Nursing Times*, **87**(7), 55–7.

Faugier, J. and Butterworth, T. (1993) *Clinical Supervision: A Position Paper*, University of Manchester.

Fish, D., Twinn, S. and Purr, B. (1990) *How to Enable Learning Through Professional Practice*, West London Press, London.

Fish, D., Twinn, S. and Purr, B (1991) *Promoting Reflection: Improving the Supervision of Practice in Health Visiting and Initial Teacher Training*, West London Institute, London.

Fish, D. and Purr, B. (1991) *An Evaluation of Practice-based Learning in Continuing Education in Nursing, Midwifery and Health Visiting*, English National Board for Nursing, Midwifery and Health Visiting, London.

Fish, D. and Twinn, S. (1997) *Quality Clinical Supervision in the Health Care Professions*, Butterworth-Heinemann, Oxford.

Fowler, J. (1996) The organization of clinical supervision within the nursing profession: A review of the literature, *Journal of Advanced Nursing*, **23**, 471–8.

Friedman, S. and Marr, J. (1995) A supervisory model of professional competence: A joint service/education initiative, *Nurse Education Today*, **15**, 239–44.

Health Visitors' Association (1994) Over-worked and under-valued, *Health Visitor*, **67**(11), 373.

Health Visitors' Association (1995) Clinical supervision, *Health Visitor*, **68**(1), 28–31.

Hawkins, P. and Shoet, R. (1992) *Supervision in the Helping Professions*, Open University Press, Milton Keynes.

Hudson, R. and Forester, S. (1996) Community practice teachers: The way forward, *Health Visitor*, **69**(4), 139–40.

Jackson, C. (1995) Clinical supervision: Coming full circle, Briefing paper, *Health Visitor*, **68**(11), 446.

Johns, C. (1993) Professional supervision, *Journal of Nursing Management*, **1**, 9–18.

Kelsey, A. and Hollingdale, P. (1996) Equal but different: Health visiting and the new curriculum, *Health Visitor*, **69**(11), 457–8.

Kohner, N. (ed.) (1994) *Clinical Supervision in Practice*, King's Fund Centre, London/BEBC, Dorset, UK.

McCormack, B. and Hopkins, E. (1995) The development of clinical leadership through supported reflective practice, *Journal of Clinical Nursing*, **4**, 161–8.

Nelms, T., Jones, J. and Gray, D. (1993) Role modelling: A method for teaching caring in nursing education, *Journal of Nursing Education*, **32**(1), 18–23.

Polit, D. and Hungler, B. (1995) *Nursing Research Principles and Methods*, 5th edition, J. B. Lippincott Co., Philadelphia.

Proctor, B. (1986) Supervision: A cooperative exercise in accountability, in Marken, M. and Payne, M. (eds) *Enabling and Ensuring*, Leicester Youth Bureau and Training in Community Work, Leicester, UK.

Robson, C. (1993) *Real World Research*, Blackwell, Oxford.

Schon, D. (1987) *Educating the Reflective Practitioner*, Jossey Bass, San Francisco.

Swain, G. (1995) *Clinical Supervision: The Principles and Process*, Health Visitors' Association, London.

Titchen, A. and Binnie, J. (1995) The art of clinical supervision, *Journal of Clinical Nursing*, **4**, 327–34.

Twinn, S. (1989) *Change and Conflict in Health Visiting Practice: Dilemmas in the Assessment of the Competence of Student Health Visitors*, Ph.D. thesis, London University Institute of Education, unpublished.

Twinn, S. (1991) Conflicting paradigms of health visiting practice: A continuing debate for professional practice, *Journal of Advanced Nursing*, **16**, 966–73.

Twinn, S. and Cowley, S. (1992) *The Principles of Health Visiting: A Re-examination*, Health Visitors' Association, London.

UKCC (1992) *Code of Professional Conduct*, UKCC, London.

UKCC (1992) *Scope of Professional Practice*, UKCC, London.

UKCC (1994) *The Future of Professional Practice: The Council's Standards for Education and Practice Following Registration*, United Kingdom Central Council for Nursing, Midwifery and Health Visiting, London.

UKCC (1996) *Position Statement on Clinical Supervision for Nursing and Health Visiting*, UKCC, London.

UKCC (1996) *PREP – The Nature of Advanced Practice: An interim Report*, UKCC, London.

White, E., Riley, E., Davies, S. and Twinn, S. (1993) *A Detailed Study of the Relationship Between Teaching, Support, Supervision and Role Modelling in the*

Clinical Areas within the Context of the Project 2000 Courses, English National Board for Nursing Midwifery and Health Visiting, London.

Zeichner, K. and Liston, D. (1987) Teaching student teachers to reflect, *Harvard Educational Review*, **57**, 23–48.

11 | Clinical supervision in district nursing

Brian Pateman

WHY CLINICAL SUPERVISION IN DISTRICT NURSING?

Throughout this book many justifications are given for some form of clinical supervision in many different branches of nursing. In the case of district nursing it seems to me there are three main reasons why clinical supervision is desirable. First, district nursing can be professionally isolating, care taking place quite literally behind closed doors. Secondly, district nursing can be stressful. Thirdly, the flattening of the traditional management hierarchy has meant that the traditional mechanisms of supervision have been eroded. Let us consider each of these in turn.

Isolated nature of district nursing

Unless district nurses arrange to work together, they will work independently. So they infrequently observe each other delivering care. The dissemination of good practice and the opportunities for correcting bad practice are therefore restricted. The advantage of being able to make mistakes in private away from the immediate gaze of one's peers, may be appealing, as it avoids the stress of appearing inadequate in front of one's colleagues. (Although this may not stand up to close ethical scrutiny.) However, isolated independent practice can lead to a feeling of inadequacy in one's abilities. A feeling of being out-of-date with current thinking and deskilled in comparison with other colleagues can result from an over-critical self-assessment, as we notice our faults rather than strengths. Lack of confidence that one's practice will stand up to investigation needs rectifying as soon as possible for two reasons: to prevent unnecessary stress if these fears are unfounded, and to protect patients if they are. Of perhaps even greater worry is the lack of insight into our inadequacies. We know what we know, but we do not know what we do not know. We may need others to point things out to us from time to time. 'Super-vision' is needed; super practice is the goal for which we require vision and insight into our practice. This may only be achieved by seeking the opinion of another.

The independent nature of district nursing practice means that keeping abreast of current developments can be difficult. Even though daily meeting with the rest of the team may take place, the emphasis is often on urgent rather than important matters. District nurses, perhaps rightly so, tend to place high priority on the needs of patients who need care now rather than attending meetings which may possible improve patient care in the future. Performance, and quality indicators which concentrate on quantity rather than quality of care, exacerbate the situation. It would seem to be important to cultivate a culture which encourages district nurses to invest time and effort in development, rather than just 'getting through the work', as this will facilitate acquisition of up-to-date knowledge and skills needed to provide good quality care. Those district nurse cultures which do not recognize this need will stagnate. It is tempting to place all the blame on management or organizational structures for developing a culture that is obsessed with immediacy. However, nurses themselves can create such a culture, for example by playing the diary game, looking over the shoulder to make sure that a colleague's diary does not contain less visits than yours. Considerable peer pressure can be put on nurses to distribute patient care equally. Investing time in the future should not be seen as personal choice, something to be done in 'free' time, after all the 'real' work is completed. District nurses should make sure they have representation at study days and meetings through supporting colleagues' attendance, releasing them from immediate matters so that they can attend to important matters.

Stress in district nursing

District nursing, in common with nursing in any area, is subject to stress. Low staffing levels, frequent change and the emotive nature of the job are examples of stressors frequently quoted throughout all fields of nursing. Palsson and Norberg (1995) have identified common stressors reported by Swedish district nurses in clinical supervision sessions (see Table 11.1). Many of these were emotional stressors which appear to be related to the closeness of the district nurse–patient relationship and professional isolation.

There was also evidence that district nurses experienced problems in the home care of seriously ill patients. All nurses, wherever they work, can experience the frustration and emotional anxiety associated with caring for the sick, particularly the long-term ill and dying. As a large proportion

Table 11.1 Common stressors reported by Swedish district nurses in clinical supervision sessions (Palsson and Norberg, 1995)

- Coming too close to the patient
- Keeping and restoring patient's hope
- Conflicting opinions
- Feeling powerless
- Meeting unrealistic demands
- Patients' trust in alternative medicine
- Feeling disgust, shame and guilt
- Relations to patients' families
- Communication gaps

of district nurses' work is involved in caring for the chronic sick and dying, stress is inevitable. Emotional stress is increased by one of the great joys of district nursing, getting very close to your patients. District nurses frequently become intertwined with the distress felt by the family and are often seen as a strong person upon which the family can pour out their worries and fears. Undertaking the role of strong person restricts the nurse's ability to express her own anxiety, causing emotional stress to build up. Palsson and Norberg noted this in their study and say of district nurses, 'They must not only serve as containers for patients' emotional strain, but they also have to support relatives in their anxiety' (Palsson and Norberg, 1995). Some form of emotional support is therefore required for nurses working at the 'coalface' of care.

Flattening of the management hierarchy

Following the rationalization and reorganization of health care which has taken place over the past few years in the UK, the traditional clinical manager functions of supervision and support have been eroded, and district nurses find themselves in a more collegiate structure often managed by a non-nurse.

This has resulted in nurses being more accountable and in control of their own practice than ever before. The UKCC *Code of Professional Conduct* and the *Scope of Professional Practice* (UKCC, 1992a; 1992b) clearly state that the nurse is responsible for not only their own practice but also the parameters of that practice. The excessive bureaucracy associated with extended roles is now a thing of the past, as it hampered rather than ensured safe innovative practice. Nurses now have greater autonomy, but alongside this is added responsibility to ensure patients are protected.

This increase in professional self-determination is a change which has brought mixed blessings. Whilst welcoming the challenges of this change, the associated responsibilities can be daunting. Subservience after all can be very comfortable; it reduces the need to think and relieves some of the responsibility for actions. The ability to extend one's role into new areas of care based on perceived need without nursing management restrictions is welcoming, but there may be concerns regarding competency to undertake new roles. In some cases, nurses may be coerced into abandoning what they feel they should be doing to satisfy purchaser requirements. It should be noted that there is a difference between management and purchasing. Purchasers are concerned with buying a product. Managers are concerned with managing the whole system. A nurse employed by an individual or organization which is functioning mainly as a purchaser (even though they may think they are managing) increases the need for self-management. Self-management, although liberating can be highly stressful, particularly in community nursing where nurses are practising more independently. Some form of peer support or mentorship is desperately needed in these situations. To have someone to share concerns with is very supporting in what can be a very lonely position, even if they simply confirm that you are doing OK or give the confidence that your concerns are valid.

Conclusion: Why do we need clinical supervision in district nursing?

Clinical supervision has the potential to solve the problems related to professional isolation, stress and the flattening of the traditional management hierarchy. It has the potential to support and develop the professional practice of district nurses. The King's Fund Centre (Kohner, 1994) believes clinical supervision is a way of providing support to nurses whilst building both confidence and competence. They state that:

> 'While the purpose of clinical supervision is most appropriately expressed in terms of benefit to the individual nurse, there are also benefits for the organisation and the service.'

How the three elements of clinical supervision suggested by Proctor (1992) could be applied to district nursing is outlined in Table 11.2.

HISTORY OF SUPERVISION IN DISTRICT NURSING

District nursing became a national service in the UK when Queen Victoria donated a large proportion of her Jubilee celebration funds in 1887 to the setting up of a training and registration body, the Queen's Nursing Institute (QNI). QNI training was often task-focused and procedural. There were inflexible rules to follow when performing procedures such as bed bathing, dressing wounds, injections, etc. The training was seen to be of a high standard and led to the development of good standards of practice in

Table 11.2 Examples of the diversity and benefit of clinical supervision in district nursing

Formative:	Restorative:	Normative:
Developing skills, knowledge and attitudes	Support	Professional and quality
(Identifying developmental needs and assisting professional development)	Time out, e.g. time to 'wash' off the 'dirt and grime' (emotional stressors) accumulated in the process of work (in work's time)	Identifying boundaries of role, e.g. • multi-skilling • competence • needs of clients and employers
Clinical procedures, e.g. • prescribing • dressing selection • health education	Confirmation of action, e.g. • retrospective support for action taken • prospective seeking approval of intended strategy	Fitness to practice, e.g. • safe practice • doing no harm
Management, e.g. • delegating • priority-setting • care-planning • teamwork • self-management • marketing	Sharing, e.g. success, failures and distress Therapeutic talking, e.g. getting it off your chest	Audit of practice Working towards high standards of care Working within code of professional conduct and guidelines for professional practice (EKCC, 1996)
Interpersonal skills/ communication e.g. • dealing with aggression • supporting bereaved and distressed • dissemination of good practice	Solidarity: • you are not alone • affirmation that beliefs are justified or not Active support: • suggesting alternative solutions • confirming nothing can be done	Awareness of, and confirming to local and national rules and legislation

the community at a time when resources were not only poor but often non-existent. Often improvization was essential; nurses were faced with the problem of attempting to deliver high quality nursing care totally unsupported by materials which modern district nursing takes for granted, such as social services and pre-packed sterile dressings and instruments. Procedures in the patient's home were carried out with what the nurse could either carry herself or borrow from the patient. Chairs became backrests, biscuit tins when placed in ovens became autoclaves to sterilize the dressings, and instruments were boiled in pans. Queen's nurses will often recall being taught how to fold old newspaper to make disposal bags. Despite this 'makeshift' approach, high standards of technical competence were ensured by adherence to set procedures which could be observed by district nurse supervisors during inspection rounds.

With the creation of the National Health Service in 1948 the provision of a district nursing service became a statutory duty of local authorities. However, in 1959, although they continued to train, the responsibility for training and registering district nurses was transferred to a governmental body, the Panel of Assessors. The model of supervision started by the QNI of checking for adherence to set procedures and inspection rounds continued. In 1970 *Management Structure in the Local Authorities Nursing Services* (DHSS, 1970) suggested that nurses in the community should have a hospital-type management structure. As a result, the nursing officer grade in district nursing was created. By this time, there was an increasing dissatisfaction with inflexible procedures for clinical tasks, and there was a move away from procedures to principles of practice. An example of a principle would be Aseptic Technique, the actual technique employed by a nurse being unimportant, as long as asepsis was maintained. Many nursing officers still continued to perform supervision rounds, but at most this would most likely be an annual event. The shift towards clinical principles also heralded a shift towards district nurses being accountable for their own practice, which was to gather momentum over the next two decades culminating with the publication of *The Scope of Professional Practice* (UKCC, 1992b). Nurses no longer had to be 'policed', but were expected to be autonomous accountable practitioners. A significant point in this change was the mid-1980s. Following the Griffiths reorganization of the NHS in 1983, which introduced the concept of general management, and the publication of the Cumberledge Report (DHSS, 186) there was a reduction in the number of community managers. The function of the new managers also changed, with less involvement of managers in clinical leadership, and managers undertaking pure management. Clinical supervision was undertaken by these 'new' managers mainly in the form of Individual Performance Reviews (IPR). District nurses were becoming increasingly responsible for their own practice. Evident of self-assessment, performance indicators and learning needs would be prepared for the IPR session mainly by the nurse herself. These 'new' nurse managers no longer had to have a clinical leadership and were often appointed to manage all the community nurses in a socio-geographical 'neighbourhood' or 'locality'. This meant that a district nurses manager might not be a district nurse or even a nurse. Many health authorities found the lack of clinical leadership to be unsatisfactory and as a result started to identify 'clinical facilitators' or 'professional' advisors. These clinical leaders are usually experienced district nurses who continue to hold a caseload, increasing both their credibility and empathy. The role of these facilitators varied from area to area, but the major part of their role is clinical supervision. The 1990 NHS and Community Care Act has further confused the management and leadership of district nurses. There are now many different models of district nurse management throughout the country. Clinical supervision as a concept, with its flexibility to adapt to local needs and structures, seems to fit the needs of district nurses in the 1990s.

'DOING' CLINICAL SUPERVISION

There are several ways of 'doing' clinical supervision. Clinical supervision is not like a procedure that can be adopted, it is more like a philosophy which underpins and gives direction to a whole series of actions. Therefore an 'eclectic' approach, where several methods are utilized, seems to be more appropriate than adopting a single approach, as it is unlikely that all the clinical supervision needs can be met by a single method. To prevent confusion and aid communication, it is important that there is an adopted or official strategy of clinical supervision which fits the local needs of the practitioners and their practice. However, this does not prevent individuals and groups getting together to form functional peer or clinical support groups which may link into the 'official' clinical supervision mechanism. The converse should also occur. For example, the 'official' mission statements, quality assurance, etc., should link into clinical supervision strategy. If drawn diagrammatically, clinical supervision should look like an interlinked web rather than a flow chart.

Given that there are many methods of doing clinical supervision, it is important that the method chosen reflects local needs. During the planning and implementing stages of clinical supervision as many persons should be consulted as possible. Ideally, the chosen method should arise out of a series of planning, supportive and evaluative workshops. The main methods of doing clinical supervision, which can be further subdivided, are listed in Table 11.3. Each method of clinical supervision has particular advantages and disadvantages; there is no single ideal way.

Table 11.3 Common ways of organizing clinical supervision (Houston, 1990)

- Regular one-to-one sessions (with an expert from your own discipline)
- Regular one-to-one sessions (with a supervisor from a different discipline)
- One-to-one peer supervision (with people of a similar grade and expertise)
- Group supervision (shared supervision by teams)
- Network supervision (a group of people with similar expertise and interests who do not necessarily work together on a day-to-day basis)

Let us consider each of the ways listed in Table 11.3 in turn, and consider how they may be applied to district nursing and the potential effectiveness of achieving Procter's three elements: normative, formative and restorative (Procter, 1992). The examples given are general; there are many potential variations possible within the broad headings given. It is up to the practitioners involved to identify and clarify the method that suits them, rather than blindly adopting a method of clinical supervision from a textbook. The following examples should be considered as guidelines rather than gospel. It is worth noting that this 'bottom up' approach is approved at the highest level:

'Discussions should be held at local and national level on the range and appropriateness of models of clinical supervision...' (DoH, 1993)

Network supervision

Practice nurses provide examples of networking. Throughout the country they have formed networking groups or forums, mainly out of necessity, due to the personal and previously professionally isolating nature of their work. These forums already fulfil some of the functions of clinical supervision and with development could become part of a strategy for implementing clinical supervision. District nurses should consider the potential of uni-disciplinary and also multi-disciplinary network supervision to fulfil some of their clinical supervision needs. Networking has one great advantage, the potential to really reach out. District nurses may not be fully aware of what is happening in their own trust, never mind neighbouring trusts. As community nurses increasingly work in smaller groups based around GP practices, multi-disciplinary team work may improve, but the lack of wider links has the disadvantage of being potentially incestuous and isolating. There is an increasing need to find out what is going on further afield. It is to be hoped that, even with the increasing commercial approach to health care, professionals can continue to view such sharing as professional development not as industrial secrets.

Networking is at its most effective when there is potential to 'snowball', i.e. members of a networking group pick up information at the meeting and pass on these ideas to their day-to-day colleagues, increasing the number of people who are aware, informed and consulted. Like a rolling snowball gets bigger the farther it travels in the snow, the comments and extra information from individuals can be fed back to the next meeting.

The formative function can be enhanced if there is some form of educational component built into the network meetings. This can be informal, for example nurses discussing problems and solutions, or more formal presentations, for example, invited speakers, or members of the group sharing their expertise, for example discussing case studies.

Sharing problems, ventilating long-standing grumbles to like-minded people and in return receiving support and solutions at these meetings will certainly go a long way to satisfying the restorative function of clinical supervision.

'Face saving' normative functions can be achieved by this method. Good practice can be adopted without the nurse first having to confess to less than ideal performance. It is possible to distance oneself from painful critique of one's practice. For example, it is possible to listen, or even join in conversations maintaining a 'poker face', condemning some out-of-date practice in the evening and them making some rapid changes the next day.

Network supervision has similarities with peer supervision as there is a feeling of support rather than criticism. There is a safety in meeting with like-minded people who understand and empathize the dilemmas and frustrations of the job. Networking has two great strengths: an ability to disseminate good practice and, particularly important for isolated workers, it forms an essential support system.

The major flaw with this method is that it is not personalized. Individual needs may not be identified or met. To be effective, it is dependant on regular attendance and to some extent an extrovert personality. As happens so often in groups of this nature, active members' need for supervision may not be as great as the inactive or non-members. Networking to some extent fulfils the needs of the conscientious rather than the inadequate.

To summarize, network supervision is a comfortable method because it is not targeted on individuals. However, the very individuals who require greater help can find it easy to become invisible within the group.

Group supervision

In this case, teams of people who work together share supervision in a group. A major advantage of this method is the time saved in comparison to individual supervision. it also makes sense, in that in many cases excellent practice is brought about by a team and not individuals. The anxiety of individual supervision 'being under the microscope' is reduced.

Before the legislation on manual handling, one of my colleagues in particular found difficulty moving certain patients and hoists were obtained. As you all know, it is much quicker to hump than hoist, as a result the hoists were not always used. This caused difficulties with patients and relative compliance when a nurse wished to use a hoist. It was noted that this was a source of some friction within the team and was resolved with an agreement that, if a hoist was supplied, it must be used.

Group supervision has the potential to fulfil all Procter's elements and foster team-work spirit if there is a commitment from the whole group and the ground rules are understood by all. However, as with all teams, if some members are felt to be not 'pulling their weight' it can be very destructive to the group dynamics. There is also the danger of 'pooling ignorance' – the group deciding on a course of action or having a belief which is incorrect. Having a trained facilitator who is not a member of the group and consulting experts for specialist input are possible solutions to the disadvantages outlined.

District nurses, when they think of group supervision, may immediately think of their nursing team. However, it is worth considering a wider membership of the group. Effective primary care must surely be enhanced by team work and as each member of the team is dependent on the others, even if just for referrals, it seems that there may be considerable merit in multi-disciplinary group supervision.

Peer supervision

Peer supervision has always taken place in district nursing. Although some have implemented a formal system of peer evaluation, the majority of peer evaluation in the community is informal. If you hadn't realized, it occurs every time a visit to someone else's patient takes place. Try using the last dressing pack and not ordering more, if you don't believe this! Nurses assess each other's care almost subconsciously. The feedback, however, is often negative in nature – 'Don't know why you put so and so on weekend list', 'This dressing is no good' – and the nurse who doesn't have a good set up will soon get to hear about it. Negative feedback of this nature is even more harmful if it is not given to the nurse concerned. Talking to others is simply dangerous gossip. Instead of gossip, colleagues should encourage excellence in practice by facilitating the development of each other and giving positive feedback as often as possible.

Arguably peer supervision is better when it is two-way – it is easier to disclose delicate information with an equal if you feel as though the roles will be reversed. There is mutual benefit and a mutual contract of confidentiality. With a superior there is, in self interest, an inhibition to disclose failures, so small problems may only come to light when a major problem occurs. One of my colleagues hated motorway driving, in particular joining a motorway. He said he coped with this by not looking behind him whilst he left the slip road. He put his indicator on and slowly moved out. Peers in a supportive environment could help him with this and prevent a disaster. He may not disclose this to someone in authority if his job depended upon him being able to drive.

If you are going to implement peer supervision, some sort of training is essential. At the very least, ground rules need clarification. It is so easy to slip into helper and helped roles rather than equals. You need also to avoid negative or threatening feedback. Avoid statements like 'I always do' or 'You should have', instead try 'I had a similar problem' or 'Have you considered'.

Peer supervision has great potential for support and achieving Procter's restorative element of clinical supervision. However, the quality and quantity of the formative element is dependant on the knowledge and skills of the chosen peer. Choosing someone with superior knowledge and skills may seem logical, but it will upset the power balance, changing peer supervision to more a meeting between supervisor and supervisee. Peer supervision means that Procter's normative elements of clinical supervision will not meet in the traditional way, such as a manager checking up on practice. However, peer supervision has the potential to be more effective, given that bad practice in district nursing is more visible to fellow workers and peer pressure is such a powerful force. There are difficulties of achieving the normative aspects of supervision by peer supervision which will be discussed in the next section.

One-to-one supervision

The problem with all the methods mentioned so far is that they all have the danger of collusion. Bad practice can be kept quiet, hushed up. Ranks can be closed. It also puts practitioners in a very difficult situation – what do you do if someone is not up to scratch? If their practice is really bad, the action to be taken is clear. In the interests of patients, the bad practice must be disclosed to an appropriate authority. Minor and 'borderline' bad practice is more difficult. Is it fair to burden people with the added stress of whether to keep quiet or to report their colleagues' poor practice? It is easy to say where your duty lies theoretically, but more difficult in practice, when you have to run the risk of irreparably damaging friendships and working relationships. Keeping quiet about another's bad practice also implicates you as you may be called to account for omitting to prevent the bad practice.

There is perhaps a need for specially trained and designated supervisors who, in turn, are supervised. They could be expert clinical counsellors and clinical leaders. However, it could also be argued that clinical supervisors do not need to be 'experts' but they should have certain desirable qualities including credibility, facilitation, empathy and unconditional regard. There is a danger of 'turning the clock back' by reintroducing a hierarchy of supervisors, likened to nursing officers of the 1980s, with an emphasis on management rather than growth and development issues. Whether these specially trained and designated supervisors should come from your own discipline or not is an interesting question.

Having a supervisor from one's own discipline has obvious leadership and empathy advantages, but has the disadvantage of potentially perpetuating ritual practice. Tribalistic beliefs, such as DN can't take blood, HV can't give immunisations, used to be common when community nurses were segregated into isolated professional groups. Having to explain and justify your practice to an 'outsider' challenges the appropriateness of priorities and encourages a deeper reflection upon practice. if the supervisor comes from another discipline closely allied to the supervisee's there is also the possibility of greater understanding of role, which should improve multi-disciplinary working targeted to the needs of the patients rather than supporting tribalistic professionalism.

One-to-one supervision with an expert is perhaps the most effective, but it is certainly the most costly. After the initial training of supervisors, there are costs associated with supervisors and supervisees taking time away from practice, and travelling costs.

Frequency of clinical supervision sessions

Whatever method of clinical supervision is chosen there is a need to consider the frequency and content of the clinical supervision sessions.

Frequency of clinical supervision sessions depends to some extent on need, how well established the supervision system is, how comfortable the participants are and the method used. In the early stages of clinical supervision little may be achieved as ground rules, confidence and roles are established, in which case the meetings may need to be held more frequently. Once established the meetings should not be too far apart as there is a danger of losing continuity. Monthly meetings appear to be about right.

Evaluating effectiveness

The effectiveness of the clinical supervision programme needs to be subject to continuous evaluation by the participants, including self-assessment. A more summative assessment, formal assessment, will be required from time to time.

To summarise there are many different ways of 'doing' clinical supervision. The most appropriate, 'official' method is best identified by the participants themselves, supplemented by informal, more individual approaches. Certain methods of clinical supervision are potentially more effective at achieving certain aims of clinical supervision than others (see Table 11.4).

TIME PERIODS FOR CLINICAL SUPERVISION

There are basically three time periods in clinical practice that clinical supervision can focus upon: present, past and future (see Table 11.5).

Table 11.4 Guide to the potential of various methods of clinical supervision to achieve Procter's three elements of clinical supervision

	Normative	Restorative	Formative
Networking	+	+	+
Group	+ +	+ +	+ +
Peer	+ +	+ + +	+
One-to-one with an 'expert'	+ + +	+ +	+ + +

N.B. This table is based on personal observation. The intention is to demonstrate graphically that some methods achieve elements of clinical supervision easier than others. It should not be read as an endorsement of superiority. The importance of this table is to highlight the fact that certain methods have shortfalls which may require greater effort to ensure that 'true' clinical supervision is taking place. All methods are contextually dependant. For example, how well the elements in a one-to-one are achieved will depend upon supervisor and supervisee. True clinical supervision is interpreted as actively considering Procter's three elements.
Key: + Possible, + + Some, + + + Good

Live supervision

There is a long tradition of clinical supervision in district nursing of students visiting patients with them. Although costly in terms of time, observing students' practice at first-hand and the spontaneous discussion of care management issues, are extremely valuable educationally. Students, in my experience, initially tend to view these rounds as summative assessment rounds rather than tutorials and are greatly relieved that the emphasis is on development and discussion, not testing. Supervisory rounds of qualified staff have been largely discontinued as it is felt, partly, that they are not cost-effective and the present climate, which emphasizes the individual responsibility for practice, has reduced the requirement for managers to observe care directly (UKCC, 1992a; 1992b). It could be argued that, with increasing autonomy and accountability in practice, there is more need for 'live supervision' than before. District nurses, because they work 'behind closed doors', could benefit from the sharing, confirming of expertise and identification of learning needs from observing direct care. A nurse may be convinced, for example, that she is using a Doppler correctly

Table 11.5 Time periods for clinical supervision: present, past and future

- *Live* – as clinical practice takes place, for example supervision rounds, supervisor observes work of supervisee/peer
- *Reflective* – the most common method, previous events are discussed with a supervisor or presented to a group
- *Proactive* – exploration of possible choices, rehearsal situations – how to break bad news

to assess circulation and will remain convinced until she sees someone doing it differently. Live supervision, to be effective, must encompass Procter's three elements. To view live clinical supervision as simply assessment rounds devalues the effectiveness of this valuable method of professional development.

Live clinical supervision is not exclusively the direct observation of delivery of care. Discussion of a current case management remote from the actual situation could also be considered 'live'.

Reflective supervision

Reflection, or after-the-event analysis, is the most common method of clinical supervision: a nurse discusses recent experience with a supervisor or group. As memories are unreliable, it is advisable to keep a reflective diary in which incidents and thoughts are recorded, or, at very least, a list of topics to discuss at the next clinical supervision session. A case study can be presented to a group or individual supervisor for discussion. Alternatively, nurses may role-play a situation in order to gain greater understanding. The nurse could act out her role or the role of another in a particular incident. Acting the patient's part, particularly if they are distressed, aggressive, unpopular or disabled, etc., could be quite enlightening.

Proactive supervision

Forward planning for future or potential situations is an advanced form of clinical supervision. An actual or fictitious case study approach could again be used, where a nurse presents a scenario and suggests some alternatives and then opens up the case management for discussion. Alternatively, forward planning or rehearsal of difficult situations could take place, such as breaking bad news or dealing with aggression. Again, role play could be used most effectively. An example of a proactive approach which is frequently used when applying for a new position is asking a colleague to set up a mock interview in preparation for the real thing.

COSTS OF CLINICAL SUPERVISION

Clinical supervision is costly. It requires time, money and energy. Both purchasers and providers may see the value of clinical supervision as long as it is not carried out in their time. It is important, therefore, that clinical supervision costs are included in contracts and not seen as incidental. Purchasers and providers need to be made aware that rather than asking 'can we afford the luxury of clinical supervision?', they need to consider

'Can we afford not to have it?' Poor quality, out-of-date or dangerous care has many associated costs; litigation may be the most obvious, but there are many more.

CONCLUSION

These are exciting times where community nurses, in particular, may enjoy considerable professional self-determination and autonomy. Initiatives like nurse prescribing show that 'the establishment' has confidence not only in community nurses' abilities, but also in their responsibilities. The support, developmental and quality functions of clinical supervision are probably required in the community more than any other branch of nursing, due to the demanding and often professionally isolated nature of community nursing practice.

REFERENCES

DoH (1993) *A Vision for the Future: Report of the Chief Nursing Officer*, HMSO, London.

DHSS (1970) *Management Structure in the Local Authorities Nursing Services* (Mayson Report), HMSO, London.

DHSS (1986) *Neighbourhood Nursing: A Focus For Care*, HMSO, London.

Houston, G. (1990) *Supervision and Counselling*, Rochester Foundation, London.

Kohner, N. (ed.) (1994) *Clinical Supervision: An Executive Summary. Report of Work from Nursing Development Units*, King's Fund Centre, London/BEBC, Poole, Dorset, UK.

Palsson, M. and Norberg, A. (1995) District nurses' stories of difficult care episodes narrated during systematic clinical supervision sessions, *Scandinavian Journal of Caring Sciences*, **9**, 17–27.

Procter, B. (1992) On being a trainer and supervision for counselling in action, in Hawkins, P. and Shoet, R. (eds) *Supervision in the Helping Professions*, Open University Press, Milton Keynes, UK.

UKCC (1992a) *Code of Professional Conduct*, UKCC, London.

UKCC (1992b) *The Scope of Professional Practice*, UKCC, London.

Clinical supervision and community psychiatric nursing

12

Peter Wilkin

'The shade of their trees was a word of many shades
And a lamp of lightning for the poor in the dark;'
('Once it was the colour of saying', Dylan Thomas, 1938)

ILLUMINATION

It is a cold, dark December night. Underneath the light of a solitary street lamp, a man is on his hands and knees searching for something, apparently in vain. Presently, he is approached by a passer-by, who asks if he can help. The man looks up briefly and says that he has lost his wallet. 'Never mind. I'll help you find it,' says the stranger, immediately picking up on the man's despair. He joins him on all fours and proceeds to search alongside him underneath the orange glow of the lamp. After an hour has gone by, the stranger turns to the man and, exasperated, says; 'Surely we should have found it by now. Are you sure you lost your wallet just here?' 'Oh, no!' replied the man, 'I dropped it further up the street, but there's no street light up there!'

In community psychiatric nursing there are many dark, shadowy moments when we lose direction and cannot see what needs to be done. Yet looking where the light shines does not necessarily mean that you will find what you are looking for. In clinical supervision, we need someone to guide us back to the casework moment, as only then can our retrospective darkness be illuminated by the light of insight.

I must confess that the inspiration for this introductory vignette came from a man who has lit up my own lamp on many occasions; never more so than when he describes the 'hope' of the therapist 'to share with his patient in the creation of a language – a language spoken with a 'true voice' of feeling' (Hobson, 1985). For me, the exact same principle can be extrapolated to illustrate the hope of the clinical supervisor.

CONTAINMENT

Few would dispute that the role of the Community Psychiatric Nurse (CPN) is a potentially stressful one. Most of them can frequently be seen plunging into the deep end of care provision, working with vulnerable people who are suffering from both acute and enduring mental health problems. Carson *et al.* (1995) produced a list of stressors identified by CPNs themselves, which included both the frustrations of inadequate resources together with the ever-present risk of client suicide and violence. CPNs are beginning to realize and accept that they need looking after if they are to survive the rigours of such a demanding profession.

Barker (1992), sage-like in his simplicity, makes us aware that supervision is 'to protect people in care from nurses and to protect nurses from themselves.' Clinical supervision should be good enough to keep nurses safe, whilst simultaneously enabling them to grow through encouraging a healthy curiosity about their clients and themselves. Although still in its infancy, clinical supervision has been hailed as the most likely vehicle to provide a containing environment for all nurse practitioners (DoH, 1993).

SELF-EXPLORATION

Fundamentally, supervision has a dualistic role within community psychiatric nursing, enabling nurses to become better practitioners whilst urging exploration of areas within themselves which might be inhibiting them in practice. The supervision setting can provide a route towards this self-awareness. The facilitation of introspection by the supervisor encourages the CPN to look inside and explore his/her own feelings. This, in turn, enables an identification of both strengths and weaknesses. As deficiencies are identified and resolved, there develops a greater personal understanding. The main advantage of self-awareness is that it reduces the likelihood of over-identification with the client. If we know the reason why we feel sad, angry or aroused, we are more able to take a step backwards and see a wider perspective of our client's problem (Burnard, 1985). Ultimately, we are more likely to empathize accurately with our client and, consequently, be more effective in our nursing interventions.

RESISTANCE

Despite all the possible advantages for both CPNs and their clients, there is still no foundation stone built into our structure which offers us the space to reflect upon and develop our practice. From a management perspective, the resistance to clinical supervision is understandable as there is still precious little research available to confirm its clinical and cost effectiveness. Resistance from CPNs themselves seems to emanate from a combination of bulging caseloads ('no time to fit supervision in') and a perpetual suspicion that such a process is a subtle way of monitoring their work by their managers. Consequently, unless extra resources are provided together with a convincing assurance that any system of clinical supervision will be CPN-friendly, a supervision culture within CPNing is unlikely to materialize.

THE ROCHDALE EXPERIENCE

Just over four years ago, Rochdale Healthcare NHS Trust made the decision to introduce a system of clinical supervision into the Community Psychiatric Nursing Service. Although there was an existing supervision culture within the team, it was an unofficial system which, despite the best of intentions, only functioned on an *ad hoc* basis. One of the first steps taken by the Psychiatric Services Manager was to interview and appointment two clinical supervisors, who would be capable of implementing a system of clinical supervision within the team, whilst also retaining some clinical input by way of a significantly reduced caseload. In September 1994, I was appointed as one of the clinical supervisors and, with assistance from all our team members and our managers, the Support and Development model was born.

The support and development model

The Support and Development model of supervision is a binary system which enables nurses to progress as practitioners whilst simultaneously offering them ongoing support. The supportive substratum of this model is dependent upon a trusting and respectful relationship between the CPN and his/her supervisor. This essential underlayer forms a bedrock which underpins the developmental journey of the CPN. Whilst such a relationship will always be asymmetrical in that there is a helper and a helped, there also needs to be a mutuality expressed through working together towards a common goal.

According to the Department of Health's enterprising document *A Vision for the Future* (DoH, 1993), clinical supervision is 'a formal process of professional support and learning'. Although the supportive element is explicit within this statement, the 'learning' component is more ambiguous and needs clarification. Kadushin (1976) identified three basic functions of clinical supervision: supportive, educative and managerial. Most recent texts agree that these three functions cover all aspects of the supervisory process. The educative function is used to describe the development of skills and knowledge, whilst the managerial task describes the 'quality control' aspect of supervision. These two functions seem to describe adequately the 'learning' component implied in the DoH definition.

More recently, Proctor (1986) has taken these three functions and expanded upon them whilst also renaming them as formative (educative), restorative (supportive) and normative (managerial). Proctor's choice of much 'softer' labels for the three functions not only has a more humanistic feel, but also helps to reduce the understandable scepticism of nurses who are inclined to interpret the managerial function as threatening and intrusive and the educative function as an attempt to send them back to school.

The supportive function

The supportive function of the Support and Development model is similar to Hawkins and Shoet's (1992) 'pit-head time': an opportunity to wash off all the emotional grime of the job. Davies (1993) picks up on this theme, believing that supervision is time for the nurses which helps to reduce emotional pain and burn-out. Whilst there is a homogeneity amongst nurses in terms of their vulnerability and need for support, there is a uniqueness relating to each separate speciality within the profession which needs to be addressed when providing clinical supervision. The most obvious anomalies in CPNing seem to be: the relative isolation of working alone in the community; the constant exposure to high expressed emotion; repeatedly encountering episodes of attempted suicide and self-harm; and the recent pressures placed upon them by government knee-jerk reactions to several highly publicized, tragic incidents involving people with mental health problems as both victims and perpetrators.

Individual supervisors need to be aware of these issues and their possible effects on CPNs. The supportive function of supervision needs to be delivered within a humanistic framework which offers the CPN a space within which he/she can feel relatively safe. This supportive component of the model is analogous to Wolff's (1971) 'being with' function within the context of psychotherapy. Within it, he identifies Truax and Carkhuff's (1967) research-based three core characteristics of 'accurate empathy', 'non- possessive warmth' and 'genuineness' as being central to the concept of 'being with'. In her 'growth and support' model, Faugier (1992) outlines the supervisor's responsibilities for certain elements present within the supervisory relationship. She, too, highlights some of the essential qualities needed by the supervisor in order to provide a safe and supportive environment for the supervisee.

Whilst individual CPNs will differ in both the level and type of support they need, the principles of providing such support are universal to all. There are certain conditions which, when present, foster the creation of a supportive climate:

- the supervisee feels safe and able to disclose;
- the supervisee feels special and valued;
- the supervisor is keen to be there;
- the supervisor is genuinely interested in the supervisee;
- the supervisor is willing and able to take responsibility in the session whenever necessary.

The developmental function

Whilst the primary focus within the supportive function is the CPN, there is a switch of emphasis within the developmental function. Although the objective is to enable the CPN to become a more skilled and effective practitioner, the ultimate beneficiary of such progress should be the client. Consequently, this function should encourage and enable the CPN to develop a deeper knowledge base and more effective nursing skills, whilst also ensuring that the quality of care provided at least meets predetermined standards. The fulcrum of all developmental supervision is the CPNs caseload, which should underpin all conversation during the supervision session. This can be divided into two sections: caseload management and individual casework.

Caseload management

Caseload management is inextricably linked to CPN casework and, as such, needs to be addressed within the supervisory setting. Far from being an imposition, caseload management forms an effective safety net by preventing CPNs from being overloaded with clients. If and when the CPN's caseload reaches the stage where no further clients can be accommodated without having to modify existing care plans or compromise client care in any way, caseload management should become a protective exercise which gives the CPN official permission to say 'no' to any further referrals until a legitimate space becomes available. Caseload management also ensures that referrals are appropriate and fit within the criteria laid down, again protecting the CPN from being inundated. It also provides a quality control check, ensuring that people with mental health problems are channelled towards the most appropriate resources and agencies available. The ultimate goal of caseload management is to ensure the best possible service delivery by the CPN to his/her clients.

Individual casework

Whilst the focus of CPN casework usually involves client–carer contact, it also includes contact with any significant other professionals, including colleagues. Whatever aspect of casework is presented by the CPN automatically determines the agenda. Once again, providing the CPN with choices as to who he/she presents in the session helps to counter any misconceptions of paternalism that the CPN may be carrying.

The supervisor's responses to the casework material presented by the CPN can be categorized under five headings. These categories are summarized below and, later in the text, the synergistic process of them working together is illustrated through a synopsis of an actual supervision session.

Teaching

Inevitably, there will be occasions when the most appropriate intervention by the supervisor will be to guide the CPN towards new knowledge in the forms of both theory and practice. Depending on the developmental level of the CPN, the supervisor can choose to do so in a very straightforward manner or, at the other end of the spectrum, in a non-directive way. Teaching the CPN can take many forms: recommending certain texts to read; role-playing clinical situations; brainstorming possible interventions; or even making quite definite suggestions. These examples constitute but a few interventions from an extensive list of possibilities.

Confrontation

Constructive criticism is a crucial component of the supervisory process. It is a necessary yet delicate art which every supervisor needs to employ in order to enable and empower the CPN. If CPNs are not challenged and encouraged to reflect on their practice, their blind spots will remain unseen and their development will be severely restricted. Ultimately, their clients will not receive the standard of care that they are entitled to. Contrary to what some people may believe, criticism can be positive and non-punitive. Perhaps it is a measure of a person's level of maturity if they feel unable to accept confrontation which is offered from within a nurturing framework.

Encouragement and reward

Each supervision session should offer the supervisor opportunities to positively reinforce some aspects of good practice. Whether it is an example of outstanding practice or something much less simple, it is important that the CPN is rewarded for his/her successes in the form of recognition and encouragement. CPNing is a tough profession and the many negatives which are encountered need to be countered and balanced with 'good' experiences. Genuine positive feedback from his/her supervisor can go a long way towards redressing the balance and making CPNs feel valued and worthwhile.

Exploration

Quite often, there needs to be some travelling done through casework material to set the scene for development to take place. This may involve a detailed history of the CPN's client or a reflective journey through a more focused episode of clinical practice. It is the supervisor's role to facilitate such exploration and, whenever necessary, to travel alongside the CPN during the difficult and sometimes anxiety-provoking journeys.

Enabling

This is, perhaps, the most complex role of the supervisor. Whilst we must never lose sight of the reciprocal relationship factor and the mutuality of exchanged conversation, the supervisor must encourage self-analysis and guide the CPN through a process which turns experience into consolidated learning. Contrary to being passive components in a system, CPNs must be continually aware of their need to forge ahead and develop their knowledge and their clinical skills (CPNA, 1985). So what exactly is the 'enabling' mechanism contained within the process of clinical supervision which promotes this 'moving forward'?

The enabling mechanism   According to Piaget (1970), progress occurs as a result of the dual process of *assimilation* and *accommodation*. Assimilation is a process which involves the incorporation of new information into our current belief systems. Sometimes, we are unable to interlock these pieces of information into our existing belief patterns and, consequently, we must moderate extant concepts to accommodate the new data. Without this process of assimilation and accommodation the enabling circuit is incomplete and growth and development is limited. In supervision, it is the recognition of the data that does not fit which provides a trigger for assimilation and accommodation to occur. It is a constant process resulting in continuous forward movement, the final pay-off being an implementation of more effective interventions with clients.

The reflective process

The developmental process within our model is dependent upon the two mechanisms of reflection and projection. All dynamic interventions by the supervisor are aimed at facilitating either a reflective or a projective response from the supervisee.

Reflection

According to Boyd and Fales (1983), reflection is a process which involves an exploration of past experiences, focusing on an 'issue of concern' which enables the individual to become more self-aware and, ultimately, changes his/her perspective on the issue. Schon (1991) created the term 'reflection-on-action' which, within the supervisory setting, involves the CPN identifying a critical incident from his/her practice and reflecting on that experience. Whilst the incident unfolds in the session through the CPN's words, it is important that he/she is in tune with the feelings that the reflection creates. Otherwise the process becomes sterile and the opportunity for self-analysis is lost. Johns and Graham (1996) believe that reflection provides the nurse practitioner with the freedom to thoroughly explore the nurse–patient encounter. Such unconstrained exploration empowers nurses to discover more about themselves and their clients, which eventually triggers the assimilation–accommodation process described earlier. These significant perceptual changes enable nurses to discover new improved ways of 'being' and 'doing' in future encounters with their clients.

Projection

In order to complete the reflective cycle, the CPN needs to make some sense out of his/her experience in order to inform future practice. The projective element of the reflective process begins to occur when the CPN starts to make future-tense statements which have hatched from their reflective embryos. Such statements usually describe potential nursing interventions, either purposefully constructed for actual implementation, or as representations of how future similar incidents could be approached. The CPN supervisor, therefore, needs to have knowledge of the reflective cycle (Gibbs, 1988) and a structured framework from which to guide the CPN through the reflective journey, for example, Johns' (1994) Model of Structured Reflection, from start to finish.

The supervision session

Joanne is a CPN within our Service who has recently joined us as a G-grade nurse. She decided to bring her client, Tom, to supervision, who has an enduring mental health problem which is exacerbated by his excessive alcohol consumption. His lifestyle is very chaotic and he seems to have neglected himself to the point where he is now at risk of serious injury or even death. He is currently a hospital in-patient following an epileptic fit which was probably alcohol-related. He was found collapsed and semi-conscious on his bathroom floor by his neighbour, who calls to check on him everyday.

Joanne is 'unsure where to go' with Tom and particularly worried about his 'high risk' status. He seems to have rejected all her attempts to help him recently and has actually told her in no uncertain terms that he has no intentions of altering his lifestyle. She is currently very relieved that Tom is in a 'safe' environment, but she is struggling to identify what she should do when he is discharged home. He has rejected all her offers of finding him more sheltered accommodation and she feels as though he is determined to resist anything that she offers him. Sometimes, she feels as though Tom is resisting her interventions purely to thwart her and that he is incredibly angry with her. However, under the circumstances, she does feel she has a reasonably good relationship with him and, on his better days, he can be quite humorous (although, more often than not, the punch lines of his jokes involve pouring ridicule upon himself).

I responded by confirming that Tom does, indeed, present as a high-risk client and that it is understandable that she feels anxious and concerned for him. Whilst trying to tune into Joanne's feelings, I also wanted to offer her further support by identifying with her anxiety. It soon became clear that Joanne had encountered some challenging and distressing situations which she had responded to in a very professional and capable manner. This, together with her determination not to 'write off' Tom as other people seemed to do, provided me with the opportunity to positively reinforce her achievements and her caring nature.

Although a relative novice CPN, Joanne seems quite at home using reflection during the supervision session. However, providing her with some structure for her reflection by enquiring about her interventions and the rationale behind them ensured that she made some progress in learning both about herself as a practitioner and her client.

Eventually, we reached the stage where we both agreed that Joanne could take more responsibility for creating a more effective care package for Tom by taking on the role of care manager. However, she was unsure where to start, as his needs are so complex. Whilst recognizing that he, himself, needed to be involved as much as possible in the creation of his care plan, I offered Joanne the use of my 'magic wand', which would enable her to create the ideal care package for him. Although this was purely an experiential exercise, it freed Joanne enough to create a blue-print of care for Tom and a baseline from which to initiate change.

Through a process of reflection and projection, Joanne had focused on her client, herself and the relationship they shared together. Whilst my own interventions had guided her through the reflective process and enabled her to formulate a strategy of nursing care, she had also analyzed her own feelings and actions: in particular, her compulsion to dash off and rescue those who are a potential risk to themselves. Her usual reaction to such people would be to by-pass the possible reasons behind such self-destructive behaviour and to concentrate hard on making them safe again. She disclosed the stomach-churning anxiety that she experienced when she knocked on Tom's door and he failed to appear. She described feelings of 'being in limbo' and 'fearing the worst'.

We looked at the anguish that 'not knowing' can generate in us and of how much easier it becomes if we can avoid those moments. Yet in CPNing, we realized, we will continue to be compromised and there is no 'real' escape route, only the mask of denial that we are inclined to hide behind when faced with such threats. This realization rekindled memories of Patrick Casement's (1985) book, in which he describes the possible therapeutic advantage of experiencing the same, intense feelings as the patient. If the therapist is unable to tolerate such feelings, they will attempt to avoid them (for example, by denying them). It is only when the therapist is willing to 'stay with' unbearable feelings (i.e. paradoxically find the 'unbearable' bearable) that he/she can communicate this strength and 'ability to survive' to the patient. This, in turn, conveys to the patient/ client that his own sense of dread may be tolerable and, consequently, increases the likelihood of him re-introjecting his projections instead of burdening the poor therapist/CPN with them.

After sharing this with Joanne, she realized that her own fear may well be a manifestation (through the defence mechanism of projective identification) of Tom's fear – in other words, his unconscious (and very successful) attempt to let Joanne know the intensity of his own fear through the impact of his reckless, 'high risk' behaviour. With this new hypothesis under her belt, she could now understand the importance of sticking with her own fearful feelings on future occasions, as opposed to turning them into a mission of mercy.

Critical incidents

Casework moments are brought to supervision for discussion by individual CPNs as 'critical incidents'. According to Gordon and Benner (1984), critical incidents provide useful information which can be used as 'exemplars' of clinical practice. We have adopted critical incidents as baselines from which to begin the reflective process within the supervisory setting. The CPN will begin with a brief summary of their critical incident and then be encouraged to expand upon it in whichever direction seems appropriate. This system of identifying critical incidents and reflecting upon them also complements the use of a reflective diary which, in turn, constitutes a vital component of Post-Registration Education and Practice (PREP) (UKCC, 1990).

Gordon and Benner (1984) provide useful guidelines on what actually constitutes a critical incident:

- an incident in which you feel your intervention really made a difference in patient outcome, either directly or indirectly (by helping other staff members);
- an incident in which there was a breakdown (i.e. things did not go as planned);

- an incident that went unusually well;
- an incident that is very ordinary and typical;
- an incident that you think captures the quintessence of what nursing is all about;
- an incident that was particularly demanding.

Although the word 'critical' may have negative connotations, the criteria quite clearly encourages the presentation of positive experiences, too. In fact, the remit is so wide that just about anything could be included in a critical incident. Whilst it may be argued that this contradicts the purpose of predetermined criteria, the concept of critical incidents overrides this issue, in that it helps the nurse to identify a specific casework moment on which to reflect. Whilst they do go on to suggest what information should be included in a critical incident, we prefer to use them almost exclusively as a summary and then use John's (1994) model of structured reflection to guide the reflective journey.

The process of clinical supervision

Whilst the Support and Development model provides both a rationale behind, and a blue-print for, clinical supervision, there still needs to be some clarification of 'what goes on' during the session itself. Although we know that casework provides the content of the session, it may be useful to identify the processes that can occur simultaneously. Hawkins and Shoet (1989) demonstrate that 'the supervision process involves two interlocking systems': that which involves the therapist–client relationship and that which addresses the relationship between therapist and supervisor.

Similarly, the CPN–client system includes the content of the casework, together with an exploration of CPN interventions and the dynamics of the CPN–client relationship. The CPN–supervisor relationship focuses on the CPN's counter-transference reactions that surface in the supervision session and examines the CPN–supervisor relationship for parallel processes which may be unconscious representations of the CPN's casework. The supervisor also attends to his/her own thoughts and feelings stimulated by discussion with the CPN, which may, when shared, provide 'reflective illumination' for the CPN.

Although this dual-matrix model seems to be all-encompassing, the authors of the model point out that it would be folly to ignore the wider perspective which includes the organizational, social and political context within which supervision is contained. Bearing in mind the responsibilities placed upon the supervisor and his/her own degree of fallibility, to supervise without access to one's own supervision would be inconsistent and irresponsible.

The contract

The literature offers us many suggested formats for a supervision contract, although the key components seem to be very similar. Basically, the supervision contract encourages a reciprocal relationship-oriented approach, whilst also outlining the boundaries and individual responsibilities of both supervisor and supervisee (Hawkins and Shoet, 1989). The Rochdale contract, hopefully, addresses the key issues whilst, simultaneously, helping to establish a baseline on which to build the supervisory alliance. It attempts to set out some basic guidelines to direct the supervision session whilst, also, stipulating jointly created ground rules between supervisor and supervisee. These include issues such as the time and frequency of supervision; confidentiality; and how the session is to be documented, together with specific responsibilities that are attached to either the supervisor or the CPN (for example, who 'ends' the session; who looks after the recording sheets, etc.).

The mandate

If clinical supervision is to be integrated into CPNing, each individual CPN team needs a mandate, or 'permission to act' from their managers. Without it, supervision could be interpreted as an optional exercise, which would diminish its credibility and effectiveness. Supervision without approved permission does not work, as it invites avoidance and may cause animosity between CPNs and their managers. However, as Butterworth (1994) affirms, it 'needs the collaboration but not the control of managers'. Our own trust offered us a mandate implicit in their decision to appoint two clinical supervisors within the team and, at a later date, through the creation of a supervision policy and guidelines.

Research and evaluation

Benner (1984) reminds us that, in our quest to make nursing a more scientific, research- based profession, we are susceptible to overlooking intuitive interventions in favour of more measurable, problem-solving methods. She reminds us of the uniqueness and richness of the knowledge which is embedded in expert clinical practice and urges us to document our nursing experiences. She goes on to say that from vague hunches and automatic responses grow conceptual clarity and, ultimately, theory that is grounded in clinical practice. However, the systematic recording of nursing practice is essential if we are to develop it and construct such theory.

Similarly, clinical supervision in CPNing needs to be continually documented, evaluated and refined in order to build the best possible engine to drive it (UKCC, 1996). To discover if supervision is an effective vehicle of support and development, we need to record the supervision sessions to provide us with data that can be analyzed. Using the support and development model in Rochdale has enabled us to design a recording sheet as a means of documenting both the content and the processes of supervision sessions. The sheets abound in data and constitute an invaluable information bank from which to evaluate the supervisors' effectiveness and, also, the CPNs' clinical development.

A separate research project is planned to evaluate my effectiveness as a clinical supervisor and which will address the broad question, 'Do CPNs in Rochdale gain support and achieve development through clinical supervision?' To be able to answer this question, we need to discover what constitutes supportive interventions and which interventions facilitate clinical development. Once we have established these facts, we can then examine the efficacy of my interventions. Meanwhile, the recording sheets are providing us with enough data to measure the quality of CPN interventions. This allows us to identify strengths which can be positively reinforced and, also, deficiencies which need to be attended to and improved.

From comprehensive notes made during the supervision session by the supervisor, the various sections of the recording sheet are filled in afterwards, including any identified objectives which have surfaced. The sheet is then passed on to the supervisee for his/her comments, which will be discussed at the next planned supervision session and the objectives evaluated. The CPN then has the choice of bringing the curtain down on this particular script or, alternatively, opening a new scene if he/she needs to.

We have come to realize that standards are valuable components of the evaluation procedure and, also, effective tools for measuring the quality of systems of supervision. According to Hancock and Young (1992), standards are 'quality promises' which provide measurable baselines from which to identify areas of high or low performance levels, training needs and resource deficiencies. They are also useful signposts for pointing out potential areas of research. Within the supervisory process, realistic and attainable standards, when audited on a regular basis, can contribute significantly to the development of a quality system of clinical supervision.

SUMMARY

Supervision is a dynamic, interpersonally focused experience which promotes the development of therapeutic proficiency. Its primary objective must be to ensure that the quality of our nursing interventions consistently reaches the highest possible standard in relation to the client's needs. Surely, we owe it to our clients in the community to provide the best possible service to them? That must involve scrutinizing and evaluating our actions. It would, however, be tremendously conceited of us to think that we could effectively evaluate our own interventions in a totally objective manner. Clinical supervision provides CPNs with an ideal medium for improving and developing their practice (Kohner, 1994). It can also demonstrate our credibility to those who purchase our interventions and serve as a source of reassurance to those who receive them.

It is essential that we view clinical supervision in a facilitative context as opposed to being somewhat of an imposition. Supervision should be an unshackling process – an opening of previously locked doors. Far from being a corrective experience which conjures up images of brandished canes and books stuffed down trousers, it needs to be seen as an exploratory relationship in an environment which aids development and promotes change. It should not be an invasion of inner privacy but a much more tentative and empathic exercise. It should be non-threatening enough to ensure participation, yet challenging and stimulating enough to encourage exploration.

Finally, we would not be looking after ourselves as we should if we allowed ourselves to be frequently consumed by the stresses that we encounter whilst carrying out the job. Sharing these stressful feelings in supervision can release personal tension whilst, concurrently, identifying ways of counteracting stressful situations. If we never considered the emotions created within us by client contact, we would learn very little about what it is that makes us as individuals tick. Nor would we be able to confront our own neuroses and develop healthier and more helpful ways of responding to our clients.

Clinical supervision in CPNing is about sharing casework moments in a common light within a trusting relationship. It sometimes involves adjusting the lamp to light up the shadowy bits that the CPN is unable to see. It can, on occasions, mean anxiously sitting together in the dark amidst a power failure of ideas and 'not knowing'. Staying with such experiences and facing our own internal distress only serves to strengthen the empathic bond between ourselves and our supervisees. As Winnicott (1971) says: 'If only we can wait the patient arrives at understanding creatively'. And so, too, the supervisee.

'Be near me when the light is low,
When the blood creeps, and the nerves prick
And tingle; and the heart is sick,
And all the wheels of Being slow.'
('In Memoriam', Alfred, Lord Tennyson, 1850)

REFERENCES

Barker, P. (1992) Psychiatric nursing, in Butterworth, T. and Faugier, J. (eds) *Clinical Supervision and Mentorship in Nursing*, Chapman & Hall, London.

Benner, P. (ed.) (1984) *From Novice to Expert: Excellence and Power in Clinical Nursing Practice*, Addison-Wesley, California.

Boyd, E. M. and Fales, A. W. (1983) Reflective learning: Key to learning from experience, *Journal of Humanistic Psychology*, **23**(2), 99–117.

Burnard, P. (1985) Learning Human Skills: A Guide for Nurses, Heinemann, London.

Butterworth, T. (1994) Preparing to take on clinical supervision, *Nursing Standard*, **8**(52), 32–4.

Carson, J., Bartlett, H., Fagin, L., Brown, D. and Leary, J. (1995) Stress and the CPN, in Brooker, C. and White, E. (eds) *Community Psychiatric Nursing: A Research Perspective*, Vol. 3, Chapman & Hall, London.

Casement, P. (1985) *On Learning From the Patient*, Tavistock, London.

Community Psychiatric Nurses Association (CPNA) (1985) *The Clinical Responsibilities of the CPN*, CPNA Publications, London.

Davies, P. (1993) Value yourself, *Nursing Times*, **89**(4), 52.

DoH (1993) *A Vision for the Future: The Nursing, Midwifery and Health Visiting Contribution to Health and Health Care*, HMSO, London.

Faugier, J. (1992) The supervisory relationship, in Butterworth, T. and Faugier, J. (eds) op. cit.

Gibbs, G. (1988) *Learning by Doing: A Guide to Teaching and Learning Methods*, Further Education Unit, Oxford Polytechnic, Oxford.

Gordon, D. R. and Benner, P. (1984) Guidelines for recording critical incidents, in Benner, P. (ed.) (1984). op. cit.

Hancock, C. P. and Young, D. (1992) *A Practical Framework for Quality Evaluation*, Lake View Publishing, Lincolnshire, UK.

Hawkins, P. and Shoet, R. (1992) *Supervision in the Helping Professions*, Open University Press, Milton Keynes, UK.

Hobson, R. F. (1985) *Forms of Feeling: The Heart of Psychotherapy*, Tavistock, London.

Johns, C. C. (1994) Guided reflection, in Palmer, A., Burns, S. and Bulman, C. (eds) *Reflective Practice: The Growth of the Professional Practitioner*, Blackwell Scientific Publications, Oxford.

Johns, C. C. and Graham, J. (1996) Using a reflective model of nursing and guided reflection, *Nursing Standard*, **2**(11), 34–8.

Kadushin, A. (1976) *Supervision in Social Work*, Columbia University Press, New York.

Kohner, N. (1994) *Clinical Supervision: An Executive Summary*, King's Fund Centre, London/BEBC, Dorset, UK.

Piaget, J. (1970) *Structuralism*, Basic Books, New York.

Proctor, B. (1986) Supervision: A co-operative exercise in accountability, in Marken, M. and Payne, M. (eds) *Enabling and Ensuring: Supervision in Practice*, National Youth Bureau, Leicester, UK.

Schon, D. A. (1991) *The Reflective Practitioner: How Professionals Think in Action*, Arena, Hampshire, UK.

Truax, C. B. and Carkhuff, R. R. (1967) *Toward Effective Counselling and Psychotherapy: Training and Practice*, Aldine, Chicago.

UKCC (1990) *The Report of the Post-registration Education and Practice Project*, UKCC, London.

UKCC (1996) *Position Statement on Clinical Supervision for Nursing and Health Visiting*, UKCC, London.

Winnicott, D. W. (1971) *Playing and Reality*, Tavistock, London.

Wolff, H. H. (1971) The therapeutic and developmental functions of psychotherapy, *British Journal of Medical Psychology* **44**, 117–30.

Modelling excellence: the role of the consultant nurse

13

Steve Wright

INTRODUCTION: WHO IS THE CONSULTANT?

Many occupations use the term 'consultant', usually to signify a person who has acquired specialist knowledge and skills and to whom others refer for advice. Within the sphere of health care, however, the title until recently has been almost exclusively the province of doctors. The terms 'consultant nurse' or 'nurse consultant' seem now to be commonplace in both the public and independent sectors of health care. The notion of a nurse achieving a consultant level of expertise was embodied in recent thinking about the nature of advanced nursing practice and the clinical career structure for nurses (UKCC, 1996).

It could be argued that when nurses attach such a title to their role, it is an attempt to take on board some of the aura of the power and status of medicine. Hostility from both nurses and doctors might be expected as a result. On the other hand, there appears to be no reason for a word to be monopolized by one discipline. In recent years, a growing number of nurses (an increase in part fuelled by the changes in the structure and values of the National Health Service, affecting many nurses in management and staff development posts) have offered their expertise, usually working privately as individuals or as part of larger companies and associations (Cole, 1997). Puetz and Shinn (1997) believe that the business environment of the 1990s is 'fertile territory for consultants' and 'as organisations decrease the number of workers on the payroll, replacement of employee talent often comes in the form of consultation as organisations outsource tasks, projects, or functions'. Puetz and Shinn refer to the experience of nurses in the USA, but, according to Cole's report, a similar phenomenon has occurred in the UK. Consultant nurses may work in a wide range of settings and deal with a variety of issues in health care.

From setting up conferences to advising on nursing practice in a nursing home, from planning and conducting staff development programmes to advising industry, sales sectors of pharmaceutical companies, research programmes or the courts – the range of activities in which consultant nurses (and other nurses not in full time consultancy but with an element of it in their roles) are now involved is enormous. This expansion of opportunities and practices has also fuelled an ongoing debate about the nature of consultation, how the role is defined and what qualities and qualifications are necessary. As yet no clear consensus has emerged as to who is or is not the consultant nurse, and the title is given to many different roles in health-related services, while many who do not use the title would seem to match the general criteria described for consultancy (q.v.) in their day-to-day work.

Many nurses act in advisory capacity to others, but do not necessarily use the term consultant in their job title. Consultation therefore happens at many levels of nursing – nurse managers, teachers, practice development nurses, specialists, ward sisters and charge nurses; all these and more could lay claim to acting as consultants in giving advice to others on nursing. This chapter focuses on the use of consultancy to provide clinical supervision, and is concerned specifically with those who work as consultant nurses, where consultancy is their principal activity. Thus a distinction is drawn at this stage between the nurse whose work may involve some consultation work with others as part of a wider role (for example, a ward sister) and the nurse for whom consultancy is the main professional activity. This consultancy may take the form of a consultant nurse wholly employed by and working within an organization (internal consultant) or an independent consultant who is (external) contracted to carry out a specific piece of staff development work including clinical supervision.

Puetz and Shinn (1997) define consultancy quite simply as 'giving advice to others'. The advice might take the form of guidance, information, knowledge, expertise or solutions. They suggest that 'some people view consultants as problem identifiers and problems solvers' and that 'more and more consultants are being called on to serve as an extra pair of hands to accomplish a project or task that an organisation does not have the internal resources to handle'. They go on to define the role as one of facilitator, confidant, counsellor, sounding board, change agent, expert, observer, fact finder, coach, motivator, mentor and teacher. These qualities are often referred to as being necessary in the effective clinical supervisor (Hawkins and Shoet, 1992; Kohner, 1994; Palmer et al., 1994).

Caplan (1970) has identified four basic types of consultation:

1. *nurse-centred*, for example, a primary nurse seeks advice from a consultant nurse on the management of a specific patient's problem. There is advice to the nurse but no direct involvement with the patient;

2. *patient-centred*, for example, several nurses ask the consultant to work with them to manage the care of a particular patient. The advice to the nurses encompasses working with the patient as well, and becoming directly involved in care;
3. *programme-centred*, for example, planning staff development courses;
4. *administration-centred*, for example, giving advice to management on nursing policy and practice.

In practice, circumstances for the consultant nurse are rarely so clearly defined, with more than one of these models overlapping at any one time. The consultant nurse may be employed by an organization to work within it as an (internal) expert, active at many levels of the organization from developing practice at clinical level to policy development at executive level. Alternatively, they may be visiting (external) experts, independently employed and called in to advise in specific arenas on a contractual basis with a particular task or goal in mind.

Menard (1987) sees the consultant as (trained) teacher and expert in a particular speciality. Boehm (1956), however, adds that the consultant remains relatively distant from the problem – someone whose advice may be sought, but with a 'take it or leave it' quality about it as far as the recipient is concerned. Pearson (1983) and Wright (1986) have laid greater emphasis on the consultant nurse being directly involved in practice, working as a skilled change agent and educator while remaining clinically involved. They agree with Benner (1984) that the consultant nurse needs to have considerable post-graduate experience and education – at least to masters degree level. This nurse has not only become an expert in nursing practice, but has learned to work within the organization and use 'a variety of creative ways of getting around the bureaucracy' (Benner, 1984) to meet needs and achieve goals. Consultant nurse roles are often broader and more complex than can be defined by job descriptions, as the expert nurse works both formally and informally to affect practice, and may be involved in monitoring and evaluating the outcome.

Johnson *et al.* (1991) described the creation of a consultant nurse role within the NHS. The post-holder was specifically required to be a registered nurse tutor and master (in nursing) graduate as well as having other relevant qualifications and experience. The role was envisaged as a change agent who would continue the development of nurses and nursing, not least through the application of clinical supervision. The consultant worked at clinical level, was involved directly in 'hands on' practice with nurses to 'demonstrate and encourage excellence in nursing', stimulated the research and the application of findings, co-ordinated a wide range of staff development activities and acted 'as a resource person to clinical nurses and senior management as an expert in nursing practice'. This way of working within the organization, crossing many different boundaries of practice and different models of consultancy, stands in contrast to independent consultants as described, for example by Cole (1997) and a report from six consultants (*Nursing Standard*, 1997). The latter had higher levels of job insecurity, but greater freedom to chose their work, and more clearly defined roles when contracted to carry out specific work for an organization.

Apart from the level of expertise, Pearson (1983), Johnson *et al.* (1991) and Wright (1994) have identified other factors which they consider important consultant nurse qualities:

- possession of mature clinical and professional judgement;
- highly developed sense of accountability;
- articulate, both verbally and in writing;
- sensitivity and objectivity with problem-solving and decision-making skills;
- high levels of interpersonal and communication skills;
- physical and psychological stamina;
- highly developed change agency skills;
- analytical thinking abilities;
- ability to use initiative;
- awareness of self, abilities, limitations, etc.;
- high level of commitment to nurses and nursing;
- business sense and marketing skills.

When all of the above features are considered, it seems clear that the consultant nurse needs to possess a particular accumulation of knowledge and skills to equip them for their role. As 'connoisseurs' (Benner, 1984) of nursing, they have to be masters of their subject and be able to find their way through whatever system employs them to effect change in nursing. Individuals with such a level of expertise, appear to be well placed to act as role models and clinical supervisors in the development of nursing practice.

THE CONSULTANT NURSE AS CLINICAL SUPERVISOR

When consultant nurses are involved in clinical practice, a key role they can play is in helping clinical nurses reflect upon and develop their practice. This approach for the consultant nurse seems contrary to that suggested by Boehm (1956), where the consultant remains an aloof figure whose advice can be rejected or accepted without commitment of either party. There seem to be some advantages in organizations where the consultant is an employee as part of the clinical team, not least in gaining an intimate knowledge of how the organization 'ticks', in building trusting relationships with colleagues, in establishing clinical credibility and leadership, and in effecting change through 'bottom-up' techniques where the change agent participates in the milieu to be changed (Wright, 1989; Black, 1991; Johnson *et al.*, 1991). By being present with nurses in the clinical area, acting as role model for best practice, teaching, coaching and guiding, the consultant nurse appears to be well placed to help colleagues through supervision and reflection. Being grounded in the everyday work-world may have some advantages in bringing to the clinical supervisory relationship the immediacy and relevance of the nurse's practice experience. Reflection and learning can take place not only 'on' practice, where the consultant can meet separately with the supervisee to discuss critical incidents and the content of reflective diaries, but also 'in' practice as the consultant works alongside colleagues with reflection, supervision and learning becoming an almost invisible yet ongoing part of working together.

Pearson (1983) has described the role of the clinical nurse consultant who not only has responsibilities for nursing practice but who leads the teaching and supervision of the nursing team. He or she may lead the 'clinical nursing unit' (Pearson, 1983) or the 'nursing development unit' (Salvage and Wright, 1995). Functioning specifically as a teacher, staff development programmes are planned. There may be involvement in helping staff with open learning programmes, with learning contracts and with careers and personal counselling, as well as one-to-one or group clinical supervision. Thus, a whole range of strategies can be employed to create the climate of shared and continuous learning. The use of the consultant's position as a clinical leader (Wright, 1996) can be pivotal in transforming the clinical context into a place of learning, similar to the pattern identified by Orton (1980) where the ward sister/charge nurse was deemed to hold a key role in determining the learning climate. This is characterized by the presence of trusting relationships among the team, a sense of mutual support, opportunities for reflection, and freedom to enquire and use initiative.

Salvage (1990) has suggested that nursing has a great need of clinical leaders to produce climates for creativity on a mass scale in all areas of nursing. Both nurses and nursing, it is argued, as well as patients would benefit from exposure to more nurses who can demonstrate expertise and excellence in their fields. However, many nurses still seemed to be denied such opportunities. As clinical supervisory relationships are developed, there still seems to be uncertainty in practice about who should and should not act as supervisor. The benefits to be drawn from someone working with a supervisor who operates at consultancy level, with all the qualities described above, may not be equal to the experience of receiving supervision from someone with less expertise. Is being a clinical supervisor something that is open to all levels of expertise or is it something that should be reserved only for those who have achieved the level of expert nurse? If the quality of the supervisory relationship is to be maintained, do the qualities of those who supervise need to be more clearly defined? If this last challenge is met, and if it is accepted that expert nurses should be the ones to act as supervisors, this begs the question of whether or not there are sufficient nurses of this calibre at clinical level. If it is assumed that those working as experienced sisters/charge nurses, team leaders, specialists and consultants are best placed to be supervisors because of their level of expertise, then they may have to carry a heavy burden of supervision for the larger teams around them.

One way of adding to the potential pool of clinical supervisors may be to draw on the expertise of consultant nurses. They can act as supervisors to their own groups of clinical nurses, as well as other supervisors. In other words, the supervisors themselves need clinical supervision, and it may seem an appropriate use of the consultant's talents to involve them in this type of work. One case study (Wright *et al.*, 1997) describes some of the challenges of making best use of the consultant nurse's time. The study illustrates how several models of clinical supervision can operate simultaneously, and also offers guidance on issues which arise when an independent consultant nurse is brought into the organization to assist with supervision for a specific individual.

The unit concerned used group supervision where teams of nurses met regularly to reflect upon and challenge aspects of their practice. The group was facilitated by the consultant nurse who was also the designated clinical leader of this unit. While having managerial responsibility for the unit, he was also clinically involved and had a wide ranging role to develop the service. One-to-one supervision was also in place, a ward sister for example working in a reflective practice/clinical supervisory relationship with two primary nurses. The consultant nurse himself provided similar support to two other colleagues on the unit, including the ward sister. The consultant nurse identified that he, too, needed the support that being in a clinical supervisory relationship could offer. Because of the special challenges that this unit offered, the consultant nurse was supported by his organization in seeking clinical supervision from an external consultant. Indeed, it was part of the action plan for the development of the unit that it should reach out to other settings and individuals to further its goals. It was recognized that the consultant nurse who was the clinical leader of the unit might benefit from the experience of another consultant nurse outside the organization. This support extended to agreeing to funding for the work of the visiting consultant nurse.

Thus, two forms of consultancy emerged within the same unit. One related to the work of the on-site consultant with his team, the other to the role of the visiting consultant nurse. The latter illustrates the potential for using independently employed consultants in the capacity of clinical supervisors. From this experience, a number of valuable lessons had been learned. It seems that it is still unusual for independent consultant nurses to be used in this way, but it could be argued that this may become more commonplace as the need for clinical supervision expands and as more nurses find themselves working as independent practitioners. Using the external, networking model, i.e. drawing on the expertise of a consultant nurse who is not employed within the organization, but part of a wider nursing network, appears to have some benefits.

The effects of the networking supervision arrangements are the subject of ongoing evaluation at doctorate level. The interim report cited above (Wright *et al.*, 1997) gave some indication of the difficulties to be overcome and identified a number of factors to consider when using the networking model for clinical supervision:

- Considerable preparation and planning was needed to identify how an independent consultant might help. This involved clarifying both the goals of the nursing unit and its clinical leader. It was necessary to produce a clear rationale to justify how the networking model might be of particular help. This was particularly necessary as additional costs would have to be met by the organization. Puetz and Shinn (1997) point out how it is necessary to present a clear case for accessing external agents, justifying why internal resources if available could not be used. A suitable independent consultant then had to be chosen with appropriate expertise in the field, who could meet the needs of the organization and the individual supervisee. Some consultant nurses do advertise their availability, while others rely simply on an established professional reputation and word of mouth reports of their effectiveness.
- The choice of external consultant was closely related to the defined objectives of the period of supervision. These needed to be clarified by the supervisee and agreed with the supervisor. The ground rules about how the relationship should emerge had to be discussed: agreed boundaries for discussion, frequency of meetings, commitment to diary keeping, confidentiality, options for withdrawal, and so on.
- Fees, timescales and the requirements of the supervisor had to be agreed in advance. The supervisor therefore had not only to meet the requirements of the task in hand (in this case, advising on the development of a nursing unit and providing personal and professional development to the clinical leader), but also to be both available and affordable.
- Meetings had to be well planned in advance, with a strong commitment to attend. Preparation had to be seen as important as that for any other important board level meeting. Clear agendas for discussion needed to be mapped out, but time also needed to be reserved to take account of any other issues which arose.

- A suitable venue for the clinical supervision episode had to be chosen. Opportunities to work together in the clinical area were combined with time set aside for private discussion (initially two hours per month). In practice, these meetings had to be held off-site because of the risk of interruptions when supervisor and supervisee met in the clinical unit.
- The progress of clinical supervision had to monitored against agreed objectives. For example, the external consultant was to guide the supervisee through the complex process of planning the unit's first conference and, apart from ensuring the conference actually happened, this was used as a medium through which the development of the supervisee could be explored. Regular reports (verbally – monthly; in writing – six-monthly) were presented to managers. Both supervisor and supervisee kept reflective diaries which could be used as a source of monitoring results and for discussion in meetings. Debriefing sessions after each meeting were arranged to summarize what had been reflected upon and what further work was agreed.

The above safeguards helped to provide clear goals for the clinical supervisory relationship in one particular unit. It is perhaps interesting to note that one of the driving factors in this case for such detailed groundwork was the need to justify the additional expense. It might be argued that these considerations should be included in any circumstances for clinical supervision. From this example, it seems reasonable to conclude that external consultant nurses also have a role to play in developing individual practitioners through clinical supervision. How far this is used, it seems, may depend upon the availability of appropriate funds. It may be that it will only occur in particular and special circumstances as described above, but the networking model, drawing on the particular expertise of the external adviser, does seem to have some additional benefits in terms of gaining access to a wider field of professional knowledge and skills.

Some organizations may use a similar approach, but without the need for money to change hands. It may be possible to identify needs with shared interests between a number of individuals, who can then work across boundaries on a *quid pro quo* basis. Thus nurses in similar units, but in different hospitals or community teams, can set up networking supervisory relationships where each draws upon the expertise of the other. Where such arrangements are balanced, no one organization is giving more of its resources than the other, and no exchange of fees is necessary.

Consultants in nursing, whether internal or external to an organization, appear to have a role to play in clinical supervision. Black's (1991) study, for example, indicates that they can be effective catalysts for organizational change and the development of individual practitioners. The years of experience and knowledge building taken to achieve consultancy level seem to have the potential to be put to good use in the supervisory relationship. As models for excellence in practice, working in the clinical setting, they can have a significant impact on developing professional knowledge and skills and improving the quality of patient care. Much research is still to be done on defining the roles, functions and effectiveness of consultant nurses, but they offer nursing another source for clinical supervision, which can be imaginatively exploited to produce practice which is innovative, creative and patient-centred.

REFERENCES

Benner, P. (1984) *From Novice to Expert*, Addison Wesley, New York.

Black, M. (1991) *The Growth of the Tameside Nursing Development Unit*, King's Fund Centre, London.

Boehm, W. (1956) The professional relationship between consultant and consultee, *American Journal of Orthopsychiatry*, **26**, 241–8.

Caplan, G. (1970) *The Theory and Practice of Mental Health Consultation*, Basic Books, New York.

Cole, A. (1997) Nurses who mean business, *Nursing Times*, **93**(5), 38–9.

Hawkins, P. and Shoet, R. (1992) *Supervision in the Helping Professions*, Open University Press, Milton Keynes, UK.

Johnson, M., Purdy, E. and Wright, S. G. (1991) The nurse as consultant, *Nursing Standard* **5**(20), 31–6.

Kohner, N. (ed.) (1994) *Clinical Supervision in Practice*, King's Fund Centre, London/BEBC, Dorset, UK.

Menard, S. N. (1987) *The Clinical Nurse Specialist: Perspectives on Practice*, Wiley, Chichester, UK.

Nursing Standard (1997) Going it alone, *Nursing Standard*, **11**(24), 22–4.

Orton, H. (1980) *The Ward Learning Climate*, RCN, London.

Palmer, A., Burns, S. and Bulman, C. (1994) *Reflective Practice in Nursing*, Blackwell, Oxford.

Pearson, A. (1983) *The Clinical Nursing Unit* Heinemann, London.

Puetz, B. and Shinn, L. (1997) *The Nurse Consultant's Handbook*, Springer, New York.

Salvage, J. (1990) The theory and practice of the 'New Nursing', *Nursing Times*, **86**(4), 42–5.

Salvage, J. and Wright, S. G. (1995) *Nursing Development Units: A Force for Change*, Scutari, Harrow, UK.

UKCC (1996) *PREP – The Nature of Advanced Practice: An Interim Report*, UKCC, London.

Wright, S. G. (1986) *Building and Using a Model of Nursing*, Arnold, London.

Wright, S. G. (1989) *Changing Nursing Practice*, Arnold, London.

Wright, S. G. (1994) The consultant nurse: Fact or fiction, in Humphris, D. (ed.) *The Clinical Nurse Specialist*, Macmillan, London.

Wright, S. G. (1996) Unlock the leadership potential, *Nursing Management*, **3**(2), 8–10.

Wright, S. G., Elliott, M. and Scholefield, H. (1997) A networking approach to clinical supervision, *Nursing Standard* **11**(18), 39–41.

14

'Supervision for life'

Tony Butterworth and Jean Faugier

With the necessary professional framework in place it is possible to construct a model which will provide clinical supervision throughout our working lives as nurses. Given that certain preconditions are present and that sufficient time is given to allow supervision to grow, then there is no reason why this important activity could not take stronger root in nursing. This chapter provides a composite view of those elements which are central to the provision of a model of 'supervision for life'. These are: some ground rules, potential methods, room for growth and support, and a composite model.

SOME GROUND RULES

Readers will recall that in Chapter 1 some ground rules for supervision were presented and it is useful to reconsider them briefly once again:

1. Skills should be constantly re-defined and improved throughout professional life.
2. Critical debate about practice activity is a means to professional development.
3. Clinical supervision offers protection to independent and accountable practice.
4. Introduction to a process of clinical supervision should begin in professional training and education, and continue thereafter as an integral part of professional development.
5. Clinical supervision requires time and energy and is not an incidental event.

POTENTIAL METHODS

Potential methods for supervision and mentorship are based on definitions put forward by Houston (1990) and provide a useful model for presenting the ways in which clinical supervision and mentorship might be a regular activity for nurses.

- *Regular one-to-one sessions (with a supervisor from your own discipline or training establishment)* This is a situation where an experienced person can discuss with and comment upon a nurse's potential and ability to be in tune with patients. It is a well-tried device for some branches in nursing but could be developed in others to be less 'criticism focused' and more constructive and enabling as an experience.

- *Regular one-to-one sessions (with a supervisor from a different discipline)* This method may be necessary because it might be that the only person with whom one can have immediate and regular contact is from another discipline. Alternatively, a situation may arise where this individual is the one which inspires most confidence in the supervisee. There will be some inevitable 'culture clashes' and these must be recognized at the outset and discussed.

- *One-to-one peer supervision* In sessions of this sort, opportunity is given for participants to counsel each other, reflect upon practice, and take turns in being the leader for a session.

- *Group supervision (within own discipline)* There is opportunity for group supervision where nurses meet collectively and discuss their activities. Specific time may need to be identified for these sessions and it is not certain, for example, whether or not 'report giving' is the right time to do this as there are often other pressing concerns to be dealt with. It might be arranged, however, that at predetermined times, one nurse could present a patient and discuss the nursing care they are receiving with a group of other nurses of varying experience and seniority.

- *Peer group supervision* There is no reason why a peer group cannot be used to give some measure of level of performance. Case conferencing is an example in which a nurse will present a patient or a family and receive comment and feedback from peers on their performance and interventions.

- *Network supervision* This provides a system of presenting a number of one-to-one and peer supervision sessions for a shared review to a more experienced supervisor/facilitator at a 'collective session'. A system of this sort is an invaluable support where supervision is still developing as part of practice and the participants need feedback on their sessions.

The reader might be forgiven for assuming that this list provides an encouragement to nurses to spend all their time in thoughtful reflection and consequently do no work at all! This is not a recommendation we wish to make. Indeed, the hard pressed nurse will have only limited time for any new activity in their busy working day. It serves to remind us, however, that there are many ways of thinking about and providing supervision, but if we are serious about engaging in clinical supervision and mentorship, a case must be made with employers and senior staff to give enough time to it, and make it an established part of nursing work.

A MODEL OF GROWTH AND SUPPORT

The reader first met this model in Chapter 2. The model recommends a process which encourages personal and educational growth and support for clinical autonomy. Its key requirements ask certain responses from participants:

- generosity of time and spirit;
- reward through praise and encouragement;
- openness to the limitations and imperfections of both supervisor and supervisee;
- a willingness to learn (no matter how senior or experienced);
- being prepared for thought-provoking material, but remembering to offer a well-considered response;
- a need to remember our humanity – when we are touched by the joys and sorrows of others, it is necessary to maintain the dignity of others and of ourselves;
- uncompromising clinical and intellectual rigour;
- sensitivity and trust.

A COMPOSITE MODEL OF CLINICAL SUPERVISION AND MENTORSHIP

Adapting the suggested model of continuous development, a model can be demonstrated which captures the ideas expressed in this book (see Figure 14.1).

THE PREPARATION OF MENTORS AND SUPERVISORS

A special note must be made on the preparation of supervisors. Not everyone will be well suited to this task. Although there has been some work done on who makes a good supervisor, there is little clear evidence other than that which would suggest some personal characteristics which offer sensitivity in dealing with others, capacity to guide and provide focus in a positive yet non-judgemental way, experience rooted in current clinical practice and acceptance from the supervisee.

It is clear from research evidence presented in this book that the role of

Stages of professional development ⇧	Pre-registration students	Period of preceptorship following qualification	Primary practice	Advanced practice
Needs from mentors and supervisors ⇧	Mentorship and clinical teaching	Preceptorship and clinical supervision	Clinical supervision	
Providers of mentorship, preceptorship and clinical supervision ⇧	Clincal staff Mentors Educators	Experienced nurses Managers	Practitioners, advanced practitioners and nurse consultants	
Methods of provision ⇧	1. Peer group support 2. Group supervision 3. Group supervision 4. Network supervision			

Figure 14.1 A model to incorporate mentorship and clinical supervision into 'practice for life'

supervisor is of itself a stressful and demanding one. Supervisors require proper preparation for their role and equally as important, ongoing support for their work. This can be provided either through a convenor of supervisors meeting with them on an occasional basis or through the provision of a group facility so that supervisors can meet and share matters of common concern about their role and ongoing development needs.

There is nothing to prevent any of the ideas here from being drawn into nursing in its various specialist manifestations. Indeed many of them are to be found there already. To not capitalize on such beginnings would be a great waste of potential.

'When it seems that a new man or a new school has invented a new thing, it will only be found that the gifted among them have secured a firmer hold than usual of a known thing.' (Sickert)

REFERENCES

Houston, G. (1990) *Supervision and Counselling*, The Rochester Foundation, London.
UKCC (1990) *The Report of the Post-Registration Education and Practice Project*, UKCC, London.

15 | Evaluation research in clinical supervision: a case example

Tony Butterworth

It is becoming possible to identify some evaluation techniques which can assist practitioners, purchasers and providers to assess the utility and usefulness of clinical supervision and its impact on the workforce. The following matters are seen as important in auditing and monitoring clinical supervision (Butterworth and Faugier, 1994):

- defining and agreeing the agency's ground rules;
- devising and monitoring the agency's plan for implementing and sustaining clinical supervision;
- looking at the provision of education and development;
- monitoring and maintaining a list of supervisors;
- deciding on a mechanism for evaluation.

Trust Nurse Executives (Butterworth and Bishop, 1994) have suggested that it may be possible to audit clinical supervision through existing mechanisms, such as rates of sickness and absence, staff satisfaction scales, numbers of patients' complaints, retention and recruitment of staff and critical incident maps. However, it is recognized that more sophisticated tools must be developed.

At a Department of Health-funded workshop, evaluation and clinical supervision were debated at length. In a positional paper (now reprinted as an appendix to the printed conference proceedings of a major national conference in the West midlands [DoH, 1995]), a number of working principles were suggested and are represented here. Few, if any, have yet been tested in the context of clinical supervision for nurses and health visitors.

Using the component elements of clinical supervision as suggested by Proctor (1992), it is possible to offer the first steps in an evaluation strategy. These first steps seek to evaluate the core principle of clinical supervision, that of supporting staff. Progressively, work should also seek to link clinical supervision to clinical outcomes:

- *The normative component* (organizational and quality control issues): By examining data already gathered for general information purposes, a trust might find data relating to the value of clinical supervision from clinical audit, staff satisfaction scales, rates of sickness/absence and numbers of patient complaints. Assessment tools exist which might further inform this process (Cooper *et al.*, 1988).
- *The restorative component* (supportive help for professionals working constantly with stress and distress): Stress, personal well-being and support can be determined from a series of reputable survey instruments (Maslach and Jackson, 1986; Goldberg and Williams, 1988; Harris, 1989; Brown *et al.*, 1995) and their use in mental health nursing has been reported elsewhere (Carson *et al.*, 1995).
- *The formative component* (the educative component of developing skills): It is suggested that this component might be evaluated using trust-wide educational audits, live supervision on video or audio tape, *post hoc* analysis of audio or video tape recordings and *post hoc* analysis of observation notes.

ESTABLISHING A MULTI-SITE EVALUATION PROJECT

While the nursing profession was generally supportive of the implications of clinical supervision, practitioners and managers alike were properly concerned that the investment in it would be reflected in benefits both to patients and the workforce.

In March 1995 a Department of health (DoH) workshop on the use of selected assessment tools to evaluate the effectiveness of clinical supervision and mentorship was organized and presented by the authors. A number of evaluation tools were analyzed and a decision made that a national evaluation exercise would be established. Subsequently, a letter was sent from the NHS Executive to every Trust Nurse Executive inviting them to tender for pump-priming funds to help in the evaluation of models of clinical supervision. From the enthusiastic responses, 18 sites were selected which offered geographic spread and a wide variety of specialities. The Scottish Home and Health Department decided to follow the same format and join the study offering similar support to five further sites, thus enlarging the study to 23 sites across two countries.

The following aims were agreed by the DoH, Scottish Office and the project team:

1. to give an informed view on assessment tools that can be used to report on the impact of clinical supervision;

2. to report on the activities of selected experimental sites who have evaluated some elements of clinical supervision within a specified format.

It was resolved that each site should be able to offer a named site co-ordinator who would be a registered graduate nurse with some research experience and sufficient management support to drive the programme successfully.

The site co-ordinators obtained:

- required access to the workforce;
- necessary ethics committee approval to proceed;
- required evaluation data within prescribed guidelines.

Each site offered four sample cohorts:

- *Group A* (a control group), never exposed to clinical supervision but given measures twice in a nine-month period;
- *Group B* (the test group), exposed to clinical supervision and given measures three times in an 18-month period;
- *Group C* (a nested group), Group A became a third group who, after nine months, were exposed to clinical supervision and received measures nine months later;
- *Group D* (the supervisors), exposed to clinical supervision and given measures three times in an 18-month period.

Provision of clinical supervision for the 'active' group had to conform to certain characteristics:

- A written supervision contract must have been made between supervisors and supervisees.
- Defined time (not less than 45 minutes every four weeks) must have been allocated to clinical supervision in the 'active' group.
- The clinical supervision and mentorship being offered had to actively include the 'normative', 'formative' and 'restorative' requirements of the supervisee.

Demographic data were obtained on age, sex, grade and other brief views on work, including self-assessments of health, sickness and absence from each site.

Participants were assessed using standardized instruments. These were completed three times in an 18-month period (see Figure 15.1), using:

- the Minnesota Job Satisfaction Scale;
- the General Health Questionnaire;
- the Maslach Burnout Inventory;
- the Cooper Coping Skills Questionnaire;
- the Harris Nurse Stress Index.

1995
May
June   Time 1 data collection from all groups on all sites;
July   demographic data forms and individual measures
Aug. to Oct. Time 1 data analysis
Nov.   On-site interviews on six sites with individuals in receipt
Dec.   of clinical supervision and clinical supervisors

1996
Jan.
Feb.   First site questionnaire; all sites
March   Time 2 data collection from all groups on all sites;
April   demographic data forms and individual measures
May to Aug.   Time 2 data analysis
Sept.   Report writing
Oct.
Nov.   Time 3 data collection
Dec.

1997
Jan. to April Data analysis; Completion of final report

Figure 15.1 The timetable for the project

On six sites selected participants had a taped interview. These were transcribed and thematically analyzed and all participants offered case examples of the content, and outcomes and process of clinical supervision and mentorship.

This paper presents some of the findings from this research and offers some case material from the content of clinical supervision sessions.

THE PARTICIPANTS AND THEIR PROFILES

There were 586 respondents at Time 1, 504 at Time 2, and 373 at the end of 18 months. The groups of supervisors (36 per cent), supervisees (36 per cent) and controls (28 per cent) stayed well matched throughout the study.

The characteristics of respondents were as follows:

- 333 (89 per cent) were female; 40 (11 per cent) were male;
- 227 (61 per cent) worked in hospitals; 140 (38 per cent) in the community; 6 worked between the two;
- They represented a range of grades: Grade D 49; Grade E 107; Grade F 63; Grade G 95; Grad H 42; Grade I 9; Managerial 10;
- Clinical settings at baseline were: adult nursing 230; mental health 58; children's nursing 97; health visiting 34; learning disability 8.

Data suggested there are clear associations between how an individual estimates their personal physical fitness and then rate their psychological well-being. Levels of sickness and absence were lower when respondents reported better fitness levels. Staff on higher grades were found to have higher levels of personal accomplishment, increased total job satisfaction and lower stress scores. Staff from community-based centres reported lower levels of emotional exhaustion and demonstrated fewer characteristics of burnout. The things that helped staff cope best with stress at work were: talking to colleagues, peer group support, life outside work, family.

PROGRESS ON AND ISSUES ARISING FROM THE IMPLEMENTATION OF CLINICAL SUPERVISION AND MENTORSHIP

One of the two declared aims of this research was to determine and report on progress being made on the implementation of clinical supervision and mentorship. Inevitably, there are important lessons to be learned from implementing such an extensive exercise.

Data from site questionnaires were analysed in order to gauge progress on the implementation of clinical supervision. The most common models used were:

- Proctor (1992) (three dimensions: normative, formative, restorative);
- Butterworth and Faugier (1995) (growth and support model);
- Hawkins and Shoet (1992) (counselling).

In describing models, respondents often referred to structure rather than process (individual, group, network, etc.). Notes are most often used as an *aide memoire* rather than as a detailed account of the sessions. Supervision was taking 45 minutes, usually every four weeks. Group supervision appeared to need more time (1.5–2 hrs). Difficulties in finding time were frequently reported. Only two sites said that clinical supervision was in the trusts' current business plan. Five indicated it would be in the 1996–7 plans. No purchasers were asking for evidence of clinical supervision in their contracts. Sites had offered a variety of training opportunities for supervisors. Courses ranged from 6.5 days to 1 day, most commonly 2–3 days.

Evidence from this part of the study and the on-site interviews revealed a wide variety of training and opportunity for delivering clinical supervision and mentorship. Time is a critical factor in its delivery and, when times are difficult, it is often the easiest thing to sacrifice. Locating clinical supervision and mentorship in business plans has not been widely done. It appears that some employers use it as a means to declaring their credentials as good employers but the response from purchasers has thus far been disappointing.

THE LIVED EXPERIENCES OF CLINICAL SUPERVISION AND MENTORSHIP

Very few participants had previous experience of clinical supervision. Although the majority reported not being able to choose their supervisor they were free to decline the individual offered to them as a supervisor. Many interviewees described the importance of being able to 'get on' with their supervisors. The location for supervision sessions had importance; quietness, comfort and not being disturbed by others were centrally important. Some respondents reported the need to use their own time to carry out clinical supervision and many listed the importance of knowing and respecting the boundaries of their relationships, keeping to time in sessions and confidentiality of information as important.

Interviewees reported issues which covered breaking bad news, antagonistic patients, aggressive relatives, the maintenance of high level skills, organization and management issues, managing stress, an absence of support, interpersonal communications, providing cover, issues of workload, educational and training, management issues, personal development and personal problems.

THE PROCESS OF CLINICAL SUPERVISION

One of the intentions of this research was to explore the content of clinical supervision and mentorship. Understanding the content for practitioners and their employers has importance for those who invest in it. Some commentators have suggested that the process is expensive and may unwisely take up precious clinical time offering little tangible benefit to clinicians. Research can determine the basis of these misgivings.

The findings presented in this section show that the content of clinical supervision and mentorship is focused on areas of importance for both practitioners and their employing organizations. The primary areas addressed during clinical supervision and mentorship were found to be:

- *organizational and management issues*, such as dealing with changes in work practices;
- *clinical casework*, for example by reflecting on clinical experiences and learning and developing new skills as a consequence;
- *professional development*, such as career advice;

- *educational support*, by discussing how to teach and work with students;
- *confidence building*, such as affirming action taken by staff in a newly experienced clinical situations;
- *interpersonal problems*, such as developing team building and organizational development;
- *personal matters*, where staff experienced distress or personal difficulties.

In the leaner structures which characterize the management and organizational development of health care trusts, opportunities to deal substantially with organization development, which is essential to good and safe practice, are limited. There is ample evidence from this research that clinical supervision and mentorship provide that much-needed opportunity for reflection on practice, advancement of skills and that they provide a vital vehicle for support and development. Clinical supervision and mentorship are seen as supportive and developmental by an overwhelming number of participants in this study.

Experiences reported in questionnaires from all supervisees and supervisors in the project were analysed. In particular through a question which asked respondents: 'Please describe one episode from your clinical supervision which you have found to be helpful or unhelpful or an episode which sticks in your mind'. In all, 210 'episodes' were offered by respondents which provided not only illustrations of the content of clinical supervision but also the context within which it is set.

Clinical casework

The category of clinical casework covers matters which relate to discussions about clinical experiences, and learning and developing new skills as a consequence. The demand for this opportunity is overwhelming. If practitioners are to be encouraged and allowed to change their practice this appears an essential vehicle for support and action. For example:

'A nurse who had come to work in a highly specialized unit and undertook a specialist course was faced with an unusually distressing situation involving an infant and parents. This involved breaking of bad news, dealing with parents, siblings and organizing a transfer back to a hospital/home. Through clinical supervision I was able to observe how this nurse handled the situation, seeking advice and co-ordinating the whole scenario in conjunction with the multi-disciplinary staff. The nurse changed her off-duty in order to accompany the infant and family home and stayed with the family until the infant died peacefully.

The development in her ability to cope and deal with such situations and discussion regarding clinical management alternatives is to me a good example of the potential for clinical supervision.'

Organizational and management issues

Organizational and management issues were often given by respondents as examples. They gave clear evidence that clinical supervision and mentorship deal with matters central to the employer and employee. Quite often the learning experiences offered by clinical supervision and mentorship were instrumental in making positive changes for the organization; equally, sometimes they were not. For example:

'My supervisee wept. She felt that she was trying to take care of the people ("patients" on our ward) but that the ward was set up only to process them quickly and complete documentation. We were not getting to what truly mattered to the patients in our ward just doing processing and checking that we were legally covered. This made me feel better as I felt the same way. We both knew we felt the same, we were sad, frustrated and angry too. The problems continue but we feel a little less alone.'

Confidence building

For newly appointed and novitiate staff in particular and all staff in general there is a need to measure performance and share uncertainties with other experienced staff. Clinical supervision offers the opportunity to do this and there are many case examples offered by participants which describe confidence building. For example:

'I have found clinical supervision very helpful over the lats three years, working in a very stressful environment. In my current post I have had weekly supervision but without any events of particular note.

I was involved in an incident two years ago when a patient set fire to themselves. The support I received throughout the incident in supervision and in debriefing arranged by my supervisor were invaluable in enabling me to continue working in the same area. A chance to talk about myself and my weaknesses in an environment which encouraged honesty with no criticism but honest feedback helped me very much. I am a much better nurse for the humanity and interest which I received through supervision.'

Professional development

Ongoing professional development is central to quality practice. Clinical supervision provides opportunities in which clarification, advice and support on professional development can be given. Importantly, it is often within the context of clinical casework. For example:

'One particular meeting with my supervisor was very helpful for me. My supervisor had asked me if I felt I had a special relationship with my own patients as a named nurse. I answered honestly and said that I didn't treat my "named" patients any different to the rest of the patients I cared for. My supervisor found this comment interesting as she was very aware of the accountability she had when she was a named nurse; if a complaint was made by the relatives of my named patient I would be responsible and accountable.

I found this meeting a very important learning experience and I made a sustained effort whilst working on the ward to keep my patients' documentation up-to-date and discussed their social care needs with the multi-disciplinary team. I made a greater effort to form a good trusting relationship with my named patients and relatives. I stressed to them that if they have any problems, no matter how small, they could ask for help.

I would say my relationship with these patients has improved through the help from my clinical supervisor.'

Educational support

Educational support refers to the support given not only to those qualified and in practice, but also to those who are placed in the clinical environment as students. Clinical supervision offers opportunity to address matters for both. For example:

'Sometimes having students around can be stressful to some extent and to enable them to have a good, wide-range experience of our particular field can be a problem. My supervisor and myself took a session to discuss this and get a plan of action together. We put things together of our areas that would be helpful – typed out a programme of typical daily activities of that week that would be suitable for her to participate/observe and we each took each other's students to the places/activities of interest. This gives the student a fuller range of experience/interest and gives us a quick and non-demanding way of providing for the student's needs, saving much time and emotional energies. This took us only 45 minutes to put together in our supervisory session – yet has streamlined our practice in this area wonderfully.'

Personal matters

it can become difficult to disentangle life experiences which are personal and everyday work. Work may well be affected by, and in turn affect, personal problems. Clinical supervision can help to consider the boundaries between the two and help to disentangle them to some degree. For example:

'For me clinical supervision has helped me in my personal life – a family member was diagnosed with cancer. Having someone different to talk to was a great help; it enabled me to put into perspective and also separate my relative from the patients who I care for that have cancer.

Over the past few months my supervisor has had quite an ear bashing from me, having one hour a month gives you time to sound off about worries, frustrations and the good times which seem to be too few and far between. I've learnt from her experience and how to handle things better and more productively.'

Interpersonal problems

Team working and the day-to-day demands of working in high pressure environments will inevitably produce problems of working together. The means to resolving these difficulties is not always easily found. It does appear that clinical supervision offers some chance to resolving at least some interpersonal problems. For example:

'A more senior nurse was making unfair comments about my off-duty rota to me directly, which I dealt with at the time. She was also making comments about work which she had agreed that I should do, and in my absence was complaining that she couldn't find this policy or that policy and accused me of discarding them. I had thrown some out (which she had found in the bin) but these were duplicates and the same policy was filed in an alphabetical divider. I felt that she must have a grievance with me, to be so picky, but seemed to be expressing it indirectly. I was not the only one experiencing difficulties with this nurse.

My clinical supervisor and I looked at how I handled the first episode, what else I could have done, and why this nurse may be appearing picky and hostile and what I should do about it.'

THE IMPACT OF CLINICAL SUPERVISION ON THE WORKFORCE

Many employers have invested significantly in clinical supervision and mentorship. This investment has been largely an 'act of faith' as employees have responded with enthusiasm to the felt advantages which it offers.

Where resources are finite and competing demands are made on the valuable time of expert practitioners, evidence is needed to support investment.

This research offers evidence that clinical supervision and mentorship have an impact on practitioners and the way they carry out their work. Following detailed analysis of data collected at three time points over an 18-month period, it is possible to state the following with confidence:

- In the period of the study while the control group were *not* in receipt of clinical supervision/mentorship there was evidence of an increase in emotional exhaustion and depersonalization (Minnesota). After the group *received* clinical supervision/mentorship these factors stabilized and in some cases decreased.
- Supervisors themselves can be divided into two groups: one in which supervisors also receive supervision/mentorship, and another group which do not. In the group of supervisors who do not themselves receive clinical supervision, there is a trend towards increased psychological distress (GHQ).

The overwhelming reaction to the experience of clinical supervision and mentorship is a positive one from both supervisors and supervisees. From interviews and measures of attitudes to clinical supervision and mentorship there is strong evidence of support from staff. This enthusiasm must, of course, be set against the working environment of the NHS, in which there is considerable pressure on staff during their working day and therefore the opportunity for reflection and development is limited. It is inevitable that any opportunity for 'time out' will be greeted with eagerness; it is wise to use this time constructively.

Evidence from this research shows clearly that clinical supervision and mentorship has a beneficial impact on staff. In those circumstances where it has not been introduced, or indeed is withdrawn, there are measurable detrimental effects on the workforce. Good employers will invest in and support qualified staff who are in short supply and consequently retain them.

REFERENCES

Carson, J., Fagin, L. and Ritter, S. (1995) *Stress and Coping in Mental Health Nursing*, Chapman & Hall, London.

Cooper, C., Sloan, J. and Williams, S. (1988) *Occupational Stress Indicator Management Guide*, NFER-Nelson, Windsor, UK.

Brown, D., Leary, J., Carson, J., Bartlett, H. and Fagin, L. (1995) Stress and the community mental health nurse: The development of a measure, *Journal of Psychiatric and Mental Health Nursing*, **2**, 1–5.

Butterworth, T. and Bishop, V. (eds) (1994) *Clinical Supervision: A Report of the Trust Nurse Executives Workshops*, NHS Executive/HMSO, London.

Butterworth, T. and Faugier, J. (1995) *Clinical Supervision in Nursing, Midwifery and Health Visiting: A Briefing Paper*, School of Nursing Studies, University of Manchester.

DoH (1995) *Clinical Supervision*, conference proceedings from a national workshop at the National Motorcycle Museum, NHS Executive/HMSO, London.

Goldberg, D. and Williams, P. (1988) *A User's Guide to the General Health Questionnaire*, NFER-Nelson, Windsor, UK.

Harris, P. (1989) The Nurse Stress Index, *Work and Stress*, **3**(4), 335–46.

Hawkins, B. and Shoet, R. (eds) (1992) *Supervision in the Helping Professions*, Open University Press, Milton Keynes, UK.

Maslach, C. and Jackson, S. (1986) *Maslach Burnout Inventory*, Consulting Psychologists Press, California.

Procter, B. (1992) On being a trainer: Training and supervision for counselling in action, in Hawkins, B. and Shoet, R. (eds) op. cit. Open University.

Index

Page references in **bold** indicate tables or figures

Accommodation process 195
Accountability of nurses 4, 14–5
Active listening 7
Adult nursing 96, 109–10
  mentorship 97–8
  North West Regional pilot study
    100–9
  preceptorship 98–9
  reasons for supervision 97
  supervision 99–100
  supervision history 97
America *see* USA
Aspectic Technique 179
Assessors 12
Assimilation process 195
Australia 10
Auxiliary nurses 96

Beckford report (1985) 132, 136, 138
Bethlem Maudsley Nursing Stress
    Intervention Study 49–50
  discussion of 56
  method 50–3
  results 53–5, **54**
Burnout 11–12, 51, 62
  see also Stress

Care plans 73–4, **75**
Carlile report (1987) 132, 133, 144
Caseload management 193
Child abuse 132, 133, 134, 138, 146
  ideologies of 133–4
*Child Protection: Guidance for Senior
    Nurses, Health Visitors and
    Midwives and their Managers*
    (DoH) 133, 147–8

Child protection *see* Health visiting
    and child protection
Children Act (1989) 145
Children's nursing 81–2, 92
  clinical supervision 82–5
  in the community 91
  parental participation 88–91
  play 85–7
Clinical supervision
  definitions of terminology 12
  different terms for 10
  goals of 8
  ground rules 12–16, 215
  implementation 10–11
  in other countries 10
  reactions to 1–2, 8, 19
Clinical Supervision Evaluation
    Project 57–8, 221–3, **223**
  discussion 60–1
  impact of supervision on workforce
    229–30
  lived supervision experiences 225
  participants 223–4
  progress and issues arising from
    supervision implementation
    224–5
  results 58–60, **59**
  supervision process 225–8
Code of Professinal Conduct (UKCC)
    176
Collusion in supervisory relationship
    73
Communication 169
  with children 86
  supervisor and supervisee 32,
    158

Community nursing *see* Community
    psychiatric nursing; District
    nursing; Health visiting
Community Practice Teachers
    see CPTs
Community Practitioners' and Health
    Visitors' Association (CPHVA)
    161
Community psychiatric nursing
    189–90, 201–2
  resistance to supervision 190–1
  Rochdale Healthcare NHS Trust
    model 191–201
  self-exploration 190
  stress 190
  see also Psychiatric nursing
Confidence building 227
Confidentiality 168
Congruence in supervisory
    relationship 73
Consultant nurses 205–8
  as clinical supervisors 208–13
Consumer choice 40–1
Contest in supervisory relationship 73
'Continuing the Commitment' Learning
    Disability Nursing Project 113,
    128
Continuous professional development
    5, 15, 217, **218**, 227–8
  critical debate and 13
  supervisors 27–8
Contracts, supervision 200
Cooper Coping Skills Scale 51, 53, 55,
    58
Coping techniques, stress 42–3, 51
'Core' groups 142
Costs
  emotional of nursing 3
  of supervision 187–8
Counselling 9, 165, 224
CPHVA (Community Practitioners'
    and Health Visitors' Association)
    161
CPNs *see* Community psychiatric
    nursing
CPTs (Community Practice Teachers)
    154
  contribution to student supervision
    155–7
  influence on supervision process
    158–60
Critical debate 13–14

Critical friendships 162
Critical incidents 198–9
Criticism, constructive 194
Cruciform effect 42–3

Darling, L. A. 5
DCL (DeVilliers, Carson, Leary) Stress
    Scale 51, 53, **54**
Debate, critical 13–14
Department of Health 10
Diaries
  reflective 166, 198
  research 105, 108
District nursing
  costs of supervision 187–8
  elements of supervision **178, 186**
  history of supervision 177–80
  isolated nature of 174–5
  and management hierarchy 176–7
  stress in 175–6, **176**
  supervision methods and 180–5,
    180, 186
  time periods for supervision 185–7,
    186

Easer (stress coping type) 42
Education 3
  community psychiatric nurses 194
  function of supervision 28
  health visiting 155
  post-registration 5, 15
  see also Student health visitors;
    Student nurses
Emotions
  emotional costs of nursing 3
  nurse-patient relationship 45–6
Empathy 7, 68–70
Empowerment 67, 124
Enabling mechanism 195
Encouragement 26, 194
English National Board for Nurses,
    Midwives and Health Visitors
    (ENB) 4, 7, 97
Enrolled nurses 96
Environment, creating an appropriate
    44–6
Ethical issues 168
Evaluation research 49–50, 220–1
  Bethlem Maudsley Nursing Stress
    Intervention study 50–6
  Clinical Supervision Evaluation
    project 57–60, **59**, 221–9, **223**

Manchester health visitors project **164**, 166–9
North West Regional pilot study 100–9
Rochdale NHS Trust model 200–1
Eysenck Personality Questionnaire 52, 53, 54

Family care 88, 89
Feelings *see* Emotions
Formal supervision 83, 85
Formative element of clinical supervision 9, 58, **167**, **186**, 192
and district nursing **178**, 181–2
and evaluation strategy 221
Foucault, Michel 146
Freezer (stress coping type) 42

General Health Questionnaire (GHQ) 51, 53, 55, 58, 60
General nursing *see* Adult nursing
Generosity, supervisor's 25
Germany 10
'Glass head' syndrome 33
Goal-setting 32
Good Practices in Community Nursing Conference (1988) 1
Group supervision 9, 216
children's nursing 84
district nursing 182–3
health visiting 134–6, 142, 164, 165, 166, **166**
North West Regional pilot study 104
Growth and support model (supervisory relationship) 25, 192, 217
generosity 25
humanity 28–9
openness 26–7
orientation 31–2
personal nature 30
practical 31
relationship 32–3
rewarding 25–6
sensitivity 29
thoughtful and thought provoking 28
trust 33–4
uncompromising 29–30
willingness to learn 27–8
Health, Department of 10

Health promotion 154
Health visiting and child protection 132–4, 149–50
inter-agency aspects of supervision 142–4
managerial support 132–3, 136–42
peer group support 134–6, 142
supervision in a changing environment 144–9
Health visiting practice 153–4, 169–70
Manchester supervision project 163–9, **164**
supervision of qualified health visitors 160–3
supervision of student health visitors 154–60
Health Visitors' Association 144
Helping and helpfulness 67–8, 70
Heron's model of intervention analysis 105
Humanity, supervisor's 28–9
Humour 29
Individual Performance Reviews (IPR) 179
Informal supervision 83–4
Interpersonal relationships problems 229
see also Nurse-patient relationship; Supervisory relationship

Japan 10

Kelly's Personal Construct Theory 100, 103
King's Fund Centre 10, 177

Learning binds 158–9
Learning disabilities 123
changes in services 116–17, **116**
understanding 114–16
Learning disabilities nursing 113–14, 128–30
changes in approach 117
context for supervision 123–5
management and supervision 127–8
role of nurses 117–22, **120–1**, **122**
supervision process 125–7
Live supervision, district nursing 186–7, **186**

Management 9, 227
adult nursing 96
district nursing 176–7, 179–80

health visiting and child protection
132–3, 136–42, 144, 145–7, 149
increased emphasis on
managerialism 40–1
learning disabilities nursing 127–8
and supervisors 8
Manchester health visitors supervision
project 163
conclusions 169–70
evaluation and review **164**, 166–9
models of supervision 163–6
Manipulation 69
Maslach Burnout Inventory 51, 53, 55,
58
Mental health nursing *see* Community
psychiatric nursing; Psychiatric
nursing
Mentors
aspects of role 6–7, 7–8
characteristics 6
choice of 7
definition 12
preparation 217–19
see also Supervisors
Mentorship 2, 5–8, 10
adult nursing 97–8
USA 5–6
Methods of supervision 9, 180, **180**,
215–16
and children's nursing 82–5
and district nursing 181–5
and health visiting 134–42, 163–4,
166, **166**
North West Regional pilot study
102, 108
using external expertise 211–12
Minnesota Job Satisfaction Scale 52,
53, 55, 58, 60
Models of nursing 4, 41
Models of supervision
composite 217, **218**
counselling 9, 165, 224
growth and support supervisory
relationship 25–35
Proctor's 9, 57–8, 166, **167**, **186**,
192, 220–1, 224
and district nursing 177, **178**, 181,
182, 184
reflective practice 105, **105**, 224
see also Reflection
support and development 191–201,
224

Swindon Staff Support Service 61
Monitoring systems, child protection
138
Multi-disciplinary supervision 85, 91

'Named' nurses 96
Network supervision 9, 216
district nursing and 181–2
using external expertise 211–12
NHS and Community Care Act (1990)
180
NHS (National Health Service) 154,
179
Normalization principle 116
Normative element of clinical
supervision 9, 57, **167**, **178**, **186**,
192–3
and district nursing 182
and evaluation strategy 221
Nurse consultants 204–8
and supervision 208–13
Nurse Stress Index 58, 60
Nurse-parent (of sick child)
relationship 88–91
Nurse-patient relationship 3–4, 39–40
children's nursing 86
creating space 44–6
district nursing 175–6
and occupational stress 42–3
and organizational structure 40–1
and professionalism 43–4
psychiatric nursing 66, 67–70, 70–1,
77–8
Nurse-student relationship 4
Nurse-supervisor relationship *see*
Supervisory relationship
Nurses, Midwives and Health Visitors
Act (1979) 15, 43
Nurses Registration Act (1919) 81
Nursing models/theories 4, 41
Nursing officers 179
Nursing process 3–4, 41
Nursing profession 2–4

One-to-one supervision 9, 216
children's nursing 84
district nursing 184–5
health visitors 163, 164
North West Regional pilot study 108
Openness in the supervisory
relationship 26–7
Orientation of supervisor and
supervisee 31–2

Parents
  participation in care 88–9
  supervision of 90–1
  as supervisors 89–90
Paternalism 147
Patients
  impact of clinical supervision 2
  see also Nurse-patient relationship
Pearlin Mastery Scale 51, 53, 54–5
Peer supervision 8, 9, 216
  children's nursing 83, 84, 87
  district nursing 183–4
  health visiting and child protection
      134–6, 142
Personal matters 228–9
Play, hospitalized children 85–7
Post-Registration Education and
      Practice (PREP) 5, 98, 198
Power-knowledge 146, 147, 149
Praise 26
Preceptor 12
Preceptorship 10, 83, 84
  adult nursing 98–9
Preparation of Teachers, Practitioner/
  Teachers, Mentors and Supervisors
  in the context of Project 2000
  (ENB) 4–5
Primary health care teams 135, 162
Proactive supervision
  district nursing 187
  health visiting 132, 136–7
Proctor's model of clinical supervision
      9, 57–8, 166, 167, 186, 192
  district nursing and 177, 178, 181,
      182, 184
  and evaluation strategy 220–1
Professional development
  see Continuous professional
  development
Professionalism and nurse-patient
  relationships 43–4
Project 2000 5, 7
Projection element of reflection 196
Protected autonomy 14
Psychiatric nursing 49–50, 78–9
  aims of supervision in 67, 70
  Bethlem Maudsley Stress
      Intervention study 50–6
  interpersonal relationships 66–7
  nurse and care plan 71, 73–4, 75
  nurse and patient 70, 71, 77–8
      empathy and understanding
      68–70
  helping and helpfulness 67–8
  nurse and self 74–7
  nurse and supervisor 72–3
  supervisors 70
  see also Community psychiatric
      nursing
Psychotherapy 32
  supervisory relationship 21–2, 22–3

Quality assurance 40–1
Queen's Nursing Institute (QNI) 177,
      179

Reflection 108, 162
  community psychiatric nursing
      195–6
  district nursing 187
  Manchester health visitors project
      164, 165
  reflective practice model 105, 105
  strands of 157
Registered nurses 96
Relationships see Nurse-patient
  relationship; Supervisory
  relationship
Repertory grid research technique
      103–4, 104
Research see Evaluation research
Responsibility
  nurses 4, 14–15
  in supervisory relationship 108–9
Restorative element of clinical
  supervision 9, 58, 167, 178, 186,
      192
  and evaluation strategy 221
Rewards (praise and encouragement)
      25–6, 194
Rochdale Healthcare NHS Trust model
  see Support and Development
  model
Role models 159
Rosenberg Self-Esteem Scale 51, 53, 54
Royal College of Nursing 14–15

Scandinavia 10
Scope of Professional Practice
  (UKCC) 176, 179
Self determination 124, 176–7
'Self' and self awareness 32, 33, 67
  nurse and 46–7, 74–7, 190
  supervisors 26

therapeutic use of 44–6, 66, 67, 70
Sensitivity of supervisor 29
Sick children's nursing *see* Children's
nursing
Significant Others Scale 51, 53, 55
Skills
acquiring new 31, 58
redefining and improving 13
SNMAC (Standing Nurses and
Midwifery Committee) 133, 134,
138
Social support and stress 50, 61–2
see also Stress
Social work 8, 133
supervisory relationship 20–1, 23
Social workers 132, 142
Space, creating in nurse-patient
relationship 44–6
Stitch in Time (HVA) 144
Stress 11–12
community psychiatric nursing 190
district nursing 175–6, **176**
health visiting 161
management 12, 61–2
and nurse-patient relationship 42–3
research into effects of support and
supervision on 49–50, 57
Bethlem Maudsley Nursing Stress
Intervention study 50–6
Clinical Supervision Evaluation
Project 57–60, **59**, 221–9, **223**
Student district nurses 186
Student health visitors 154–5
contribution of CPTs 155–7
debriefing process 156–7
factors influencing supervision
process 158–60
Student nurses 4, 96, 97, 228
and mentorship 6, 7, 97–8
Supervisors 11, 184
best people for the role of 82
consultant nurses as 208–13
expertise needed 16
learning disabilities nursing 126
parents as in children's nursing
89–90
preparation 217–19
psychiatric nursing 70, 192, 194, 195
in social work 8
thought of as authoritarian 8
see also Supervisory relationship
Supervisory relationship 19–20

consultant nurses and 209
CPTs and student health visitors
158, 159
growth and support model 25–35,
192
managers and health visitors 138–41
in nursing 24–5
psychiatric nursing 72–3, 199
in psychotherapy 21–2, 22–3
in social work 20–1, 23
Support 167–8
health visiting 134–42, 167–8
North West Regional pilot study
109
social support and stress 50, 61–2
Support and Development model
191–2
the contract 200
critical incidents 198–9
developmental function 193–5
the mandate 200
reflective process 195–6
research and evaluation 200–1
supervision process 199
supervision session example 196–8
supportive function 192–3
Swindon Staff Support Service model
61

Teamwork 135, 168–9, 229
Training for supervisors and
supervisees 169
Trust between supervisor and
supervisee 33–4

UKCC (United Kingdom Central
Council for Nursing, Midwifery
and Health Visiting) 15, 43
and clinical supervision 1, 15, 144,
146, 147, 163, 170
Code of Professional Conduct 176
Post Registration Education and
Practice (PREP) 5, 98, 198
Scope of Professional Practice 176,
179
USA 5, 10, 19, 99

Vision of the Future, A (DoH, 1993)
81, 99, 160, 191

Ward sisters 45, 96
Winnicott, D. W. 44–5